THE FALL GUY

How to Keep Gravity from Ruining Your Day

WAYNE GRADMAN, MD

Illustrations by Jonathan Brown

It takes a child one year to acquire independent movement and ten years to acquire independent mobility. An old person can lose both in a day.

—Bernard Isaacs[1]

I know people fall down, but why do they trip up?

—An early reader of this book

To my loving wife, Susan, of more than fifty years,
who patiently picks me up each time I fall,

And my two sons, Eric and Andrew, whose talents continue
to astonish me more and more with each passing day,

And my two beautiful daughters-in-law, Jenn and Marissa,
Poets of music and kindness respectively,

And my grandson, Dash, an inquisitive and brilliant addition
to our family, who is a clone of his father and my wife,
whom he calls Gogo,

And to angelic Goldie, who recently graduated
from the NICU.

CONTENTS

CONTENTS

ACKNOWLEDGMENTS

To Bill Sloan, MD, who insisted I go the University of Chicago and not apply to the Ivies.

To my aunt Libby, who expressed shock that I would want to be a full-time medical researcher and not a treating physician,

And to the Harvard recruiter who, for different reasons, persuaded me to go to Harvard Medical School,

And to the Harvard adviser of a small group of HMS first year students after he declared that you never know what you will be ten years from then, and I emphatically responded that I knew what I would *not* be, and that was to become a surgeon,

And To Bill Silen, MD, who had been recruited from the west coast to Beth Israel Hospital's door step just days before I started my reputedly easy surgery rotation. In the course of the next three months I got up at 5 AM every day to beat him to the patients' side before he showed up at 5:30 AM to make rounds and chastise those who were reluctant to do the same. After about a month, I desperately wanted to be a surgeon like him,

And to Ernie Shore, MD, whose example of compassionate, skillful patient care informed my decision to go into vascular surgery.

I would also like to thank Elisa Alon, who lives next to the beautiful Sea of Galilee in Israel and who forwards Shabbat greetings along with a sunrise photo of the sea every week, and Joan Berger, who sat directly behind me in high school and, as I recall but she doesn't, mercilessly made fun of my hand-me-down wardrobe. She is now a retired English teacher living in my home town of Chicago. Both

ACKNOWLEDGMENTS

Elisa and Joan reviewed an early draft of my manuscript and offered invaluable advice on content and style.

Herman Pontzer, PhD, read the portion of the text dealing with diets. He also fact checked my understanding and the conclusions of his research.

Richard Silver, OD, read the chapter on cataracts and corrected the innumerable errors I made. Medical school just doesn't teach us much about the second most complex organ in our body (the brain comes first.)

Drs. Hyun Bae, Bernard Salick, Colin Stokol, Andy Schwartz, Andrew Weil, and Nicole Fram tacitly permitted the use of their names in anecdotes.

And many thanks to Andrew and Marissa Gradman for discovering the exhibit of Toscanini's shoes at the New York Public Library, and Sara Spink who forwarded a picture of them to me.

I serendipitously discovered Jonathan Brown, whose cartoon wizardry transformed my book into a fun way to teach others how to prevent falls. I hired my other collaborators either through friends (Aviva Layton for aesthetic editing), on my own (Monica O. for line-by-line editing), or through Reedsy, a company that helps authors connect with first rate professionals. With their help, I found and cherish the skills of all those who collectively allowed me to inch my way to publication for this first-time author. So thank yous also go to my developmental editor, Jonathan Todd; my designer, Brandi Avant; my publisher, Louise Newlands; my website designer and host, Steve Tu; and my marketing team—Dalyn Miller, Corinne Chee, Jimmy Dwyer, as well as Diana Breneiser, who served as my rock-star podcast booker.

INTRODUCTION

You may well ask why I fancy myself an expert on preventing falls. The simple answer is because I have extensive personal experience with them. In fact, my nickname could be über-klutz, a word that mashes the German word, *über,* meaning over-the-top, and klutz from the Yiddish word meaning a clumsy oaf. My numerous downfalls, as you will shortly see, give me more than enough street cred to promote the measures I will be recommending in this book.

I will occasionally relate a fall that is unforced—that is to say does not appear to have a potentially correctable cause, like the time I was on rollerblades just standing there minding my own business, and then spontaneously crashed to the pavement and fractured a front tooth, or the time I was on skis, standing still and waiting for my wife to join me at the bottom of the slope. I fell and fractured my shoulder. Both falls highlight the potential danger of spontaneous falls that evidently have no obvious cause. In both cases, I simply dropped to the ground with no time to formulate a strategy to land on a part of my body that would cause no damage.

Medical journals are filled with facts about falls. For example, a study[2] was published in *Preventive Medicine* that assesses the prevalence of falls (how widespread they are), factors predicting future falls, and health impacts of falls due to balance and walking problems in older adults. The authors examined baseline factors predicting falls at follow-up, and estimated the impact of falls, and balance and walking problems on the individual's health-related quality of life, mortality, and quality-adjusted life years (QALYs). The strongest predictors of falls are previous falls, balance, and walking problems. Many self-reported chronic conditions, such as depression, stroke, and diabetes, as well as common symptoms in older people, such as urinary leakage [sic] also predict falls, but to a lesser degree.* Finally they conclude that falls are associated with an increase in mortality, falls are a major problem for US elderly, and falls will continue to have a greater impact as the population ages.

Phew!

I hope you caught the irony that an article devoted to factors that lead to falls was published in *Preventive Medicine,* an article that says *nothing* about preventing falls. Even though "urinary leakage" may precede a fall, it would have been helpful if the authors had advised such individuals to turn on the lights and watch where they're walking on the way to the bathroom.

One excellent source of the medical information I relied on to write this book comes from a different academic publication published in the journal JAMA. It is titled "Risk Assessment and Prevention of Falls in Older Community-Dwelling Adults", and is written for members of the American Medical Association.[3] The article anchored my thinking about the subject of falls in general, and the elderly in particular. It includes assessment and good basic advice on how to prevent falls in people who live at home.

The article starts by dividing falls into two categories, intrinsic or extrinsic. **Intrinsic** falls are those that result from disorders such as cerebral palsy, Parkinson's disease, stroke, dementia, and bulimia,

---

*Most physicians would use the word incontinence instead of urinary leakage.

Here is my advice for getting to the bathroom in the middle of the night:

1. *Sit on the edge of the bed for a few moments to equilibrate your circulation.*

2. *If you don't have a well-lit path to the bathroom or don't have lights that automatically go on at night, get them by all means, but in the meantime, turn on suitable lights to achieve that purpose.*

3. *Follow the twenty-foot rule that I propose in chapter 1.*

which usually occurs most frequently in young female teenagers. Psychological factors also play a role in falls, chief among them is a fear of falling (common in the frail elderly).

Intrinsic risk factors are difficult to prevent or treat. I recently met a young woman who immigrated from Morocco. She was born with cerebral palsy and she falls frequently. I also recall one of my medical school classmates, Stephen Pauker, who recently passed away. He became a brilliant medical researcher with world-wide impact. He, too, had cerebral palsy, but he was one of the brightest members of my Harvard Medical School class of '68, a class that was distinguished by having one of its members, Ralph Steinman, receive the Nobel Prize for physiology in 2011 three day after he died of pancreatic cancer, ironically the same disease for which he did pioneering research to receive the Nobel Prize in the first place. As you may know, Nobel Prizes are awarded only to the living, but in this case the committee made an exception because they previously had decided Ralph was alive when they made the decision to give him the award. Our class also had Andrew Weill, who became a best seller of nutrition advice. During medical school, I never would have predicted that, since he was easily the plumpest member of our class. But as I look at his book covers over time, it appears that he has followed his own advice, and he looks thinner with each new book.

Most of the chapters of this book deal with how to prevent **extrinsic** fall factors, the kind you have more control over. To be sure, fall rates increase dramatically after age 65, but this book discusses issues of importance to all adults. I was surprised to learn that most serious home falls occur in the bedroom (22.9%), and on stairs (22.9%), followed closely by falls in the bathroom (22.7%) .

The goal of this book is to provide advice on *preventing* falls, thereby inadvertently slashing the income of my collegial brain, shoulder, and hip surgeons (they don't need the money). You will read many examples of falls that I, family members, and others have experienced and the simple measures we could have taken to prevent them.

INTRODUCTION

The black and white photographs in the book may be seen in color on the website https:/www.wgradman.com. In the header, click on *The Fall Guy,* and scroll down beneath the book excerpt.

As they say in the News in Slow Spanish podcast, "Deja que se levanten las cortinas."[†]

[†] "Let the curtains rise".

CHAPTER 1

The Twenty-Foot Rule

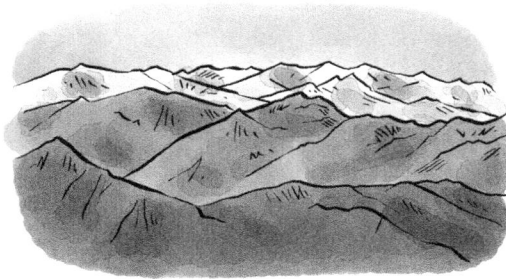

On a clear, smog-free day (rare in Los Angeles at that time), my wife Susie and I rented bikes in Santa Monica and rolled south on the Marvin Braude Bike Trail adjacent to the beach. This beautiful trail runs twenty-two miles from Will Rogers State Beach in the north down to Torrance.

On our way back, I saw a short, gentle path leading to a knoll, which turned out to be a car park. I wanted to admire the normally obscured San Gabriel, Santa Monica, and Verdugo Mountains that encircle LA.

As I biked slowly through the car park, my gaze fixed on the horizon, I didn't see a speed bump. I dropped to the pavement in slow motion and landed directly on my right knee. I heard a crack.

I immediately realized this was not a good sign. We were right near Little Company of Mary Hospital in Torrance, and before long I learned that I had fractured my right patella (kneecap) directly across the middle. Surprisingly, it didn't hurt much, and I could walk because the patella does not bear any of the body's weight.

It so happens I had scheduled surgery for a patient later that day. I reached my orthopedic surgeon, Andy Schwartz, and he was available to treat my injury at that very time. I called the operating room and switched myself out for the previously scheduled patient, made myself NPO (nothing to eat or drink), and Susie and I drove to the hospital.

Andy planned simply to remove my patella, since I didn't need it to walk. I rejected that treatment vehemently. (In high school, when I was—not for long—on the junior basketball team despite my towering five feet, eight inch height, one of the school's coeds called me Legs Gradman because of my shapely gams.) I persuaded Andy not to remove the patella but rather to bolt the sundered bone segments, which he obligingly did. I am reminded of that wise decision every time I pass through a full-body scanner at the airport.*

On our way home from the hospital Susie came up with an excellent suggestion, which I decided immediately to incorporate as a rule, namely that you should repeatedly look twenty feet ahead to determine if there are *any* lurking hazards before you. You should also pay special attention when you step on to or down from curbs.†

---

*My rejection of the proposed treatment came in handy when I once attended a concert at Disney Hall. At intermission, a good friend rushed to me because an elderly woman seated near her had fallen while going up the stairs to get to the foyer. On examination, I easily felt the fracture across her knee, the same fracture I had sustained. Paramedics were called to transfer her to a hospital, but I reassured the woman's daughter that I was confident of my diagnosis, and suggested to her that if her surgeon recommends that the patella be removed, she could inquire that if it were all the same, could the two segments be bolted together rather than be removed. After all, it's going to be surgery, and she would be out of the hospital on crutches the next day either way.

†In both Beverly Hills and Los Angeles, sidewalks are made of concrete and streets are paved with asphalt. The boundary of the two is anywhere from one to four feet in the street from the curb. At the point they meet in the street, there is a mismatch between the height of the concrete and asphalt, with the asphalt usually being slightly higher. On two occasions I stumbled

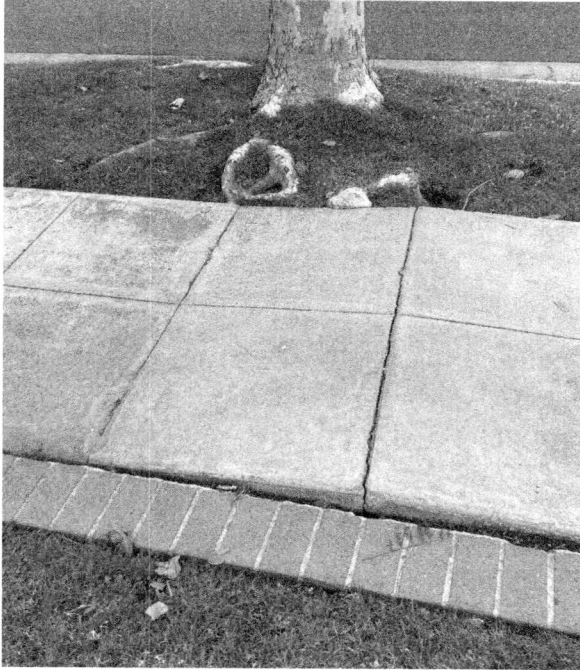

Figure 1. *Cedar tree roots often buckle the sidewalk on our block. The Public Works Department marked two areas where the sidewalk edges do not line up properly. This alerts walkers to dangerous areas and signals the repair crew where to shave the sidewalk.*

This was my introduction to the twenty-foot rule. It was my first major fall, but I would soon ramp up that number.[‡]

---

when I crossed this boundary after I stepped into the street because I instinctively tend to raise my head whenever I step down from the curb and so I don't see the mismatch.

[‡] Susie is absolutely convinced that when you cross the street at a crosswalk, you should look not only twenty feet in front you, but also in both directions to see whether cars are barreling down on you. I politely respond that the likelihood of being hit is very low and that I'm willing to take my chances. The odds are one in a 100,000 for pedestrians even if they are using a white mobility cane (mobility is the preferred word for this type of cane.) The chances of being hit by a drunk driver are about one in ten thousand. I believe that makes sense, because the vast majority of drivers, even the drunk ones, will see you and brake, even if you're blind and crossing the street using a cane.

On another fine Los Angeles day, my wife and I started on a neighborhood walk. Only steps from our home, I stumbled on a sidewalk edge pushed up less than half an inch. OK, so it was years after the day I fell off my bike and I *had* promised to follow Susie's twenty-foot rule, but I confess I wasn't following it as closely as I should. To be honest, I wasn't following it at all. I thought I only scraped the front of my right leg and X-rays showed no fracture. The ER doctor diagnosed a contusion, which is a fancy word for a bruise. Either way, I suffered excruciating pain for about six weeks.

Guideone Insurance has an excellent website enumerating the many risks sidewalks pose.[4] I live in Beverly Hills, where sidewalk maintenance is a high priority, in part because its residents and visitors are relatively well off and are far more inclined to sue the city than normal folks from normal places. When a tree root buckles the sidewalk and two slabs don't line up, the edges of each slab are promptly shaved to even them out (fig. 1). Our city's maintenance staff aggressively fixes these hazards, but they can't be everywhere. And frankly, where do you draw the line?

There are unexpected benefits to following the twenty-foot rule. Over the years, my brother-in-law Steve found hundreds of dollars of coins and bills just lying on the ground. He donates it all to the Salvation Army. I have diligently followed the twenty-foot rule ever since my fall on the sidewalk, but all I've found is a single penny, even after I fixed my cataracts. I put that penny near my computer to remind me I have at least $199.99 to go to match Steve. I remain eternally optimistic.

An important corollary to the twenty-foot rule is not to walk and look at your cellphone at the same time.[5] The reason for this recommendation is straightforward. While you are engaged in your phone, you are not checking twenty feet ahead of you for hazards. Furthermore, after you reach forty years of age, your ability to focus on objects close to you starts to deteriorate rapidly (a condition known as presbyopia), and you will eventually come to rely on glasses to read the phone. Switching between trying to read the phone with reading glasses and checking twenty feet ahead of you without them becomes an increasingly fraught endeavor (see the cover of this book).

En route to getting a COVID test at a hospital testing site, I jaywalked across a residential street while consulting Google Maps. Unsurprisingly, I tripped on the opposite curb and extended my left arm forward to brace the fall. Mercifully, I fell onto grass. Nonetheless, I experienced immediate shoulder pain, so I suspected a fracture. I proceeded to my COVID test appointment and additionally asked for a shoulder X-ray. As expected, the shoulder was fractured. Andy advised me just to wear a sling. After a few weeks, I was fine.

I wasn't so lucky the next time I fell because I was looking at Google Maps and walking at the same time. In my family, I'm known for always repeating a mistake one or more times before the lesson really sinks in. To be a klutz is one thing, but add to it my repeated failure to adhere to my wife's wise words of counsel borders on ingratitude.

On a solo visit to Italy, a personal favorite, I was staying in a lovely, ultra-modern seaside hotel in Naples. I was heading out for a gourmet fish dinner engrossed in my cellphone for directions, but the hotel elevator's bottom floor stopped at the lobby, which was one floor above the entrance to the hotel. You have to wonder why an architect would design a hotel that way. Wide stairs covered in monochromatic jet-black carpet led down from that level to the street level. The only banister was on the far right.

I stumbled and fell down the entire flight of stairs, repeatedly grasping for the banister, which lay several feet away. A polished marble floor at the bottom extended about ten feet to end in a set of floating stairs[§] that were the mirror image of the stairs I had just tumbled down. I slid across the slick floor, and my left arm, still clutching my cellphone, slipped under the opposite floating bottom stair right up to my shoulder and then jammed. I couldn't extract the arm myself,

---

[§]Floating stairs are designed to look like they're floating in midair without any structural support.

and the hotel staff had to pull up hard on the staircase to allow me to release it. I experienced intense pain. Once again I had fractured my shoulder.

The good news was that medical care in Italy is free, so I didn't have to pull out my insurance cards. The bad news was that I had to fly home for a reverse total shoulder replacement. I wish that surgery on no one, not even my worst enemy. I had never experienced anything so painful in my life.

Recovery, which included intensive physical therapy, was an agonizing three months. The stairway clearly had a design flaw. A banister running down the center might have reduced if not eliminated the consequences of my fall.

Italy has many examples of obvious building design flaws. Susie and I were on a tour of Sicily. In Palermo, we stayed at a remodeled baroque hotel that had a gigantic shower room with a highly polished marble floor but neither grab bars nor a non-slip floor mat. Susie had just taken her shower and the floor was still slick. The shower spigot was dead center on the longest wall, and I feared for my life as I inched my way to the water.

It reminded me of the time we miraculously snagged a free 2600 square foot upgrade at the Venetian Hotel in Las Vegas with an iconic blackjack table squarely in the center of the living room, but— sorry, Venetian—I have an aversion to gambling. The bathroom was proportionally distanced about fifty feet away from our bed, which

THE TWENTY-FOOT RULE

Look ahead of you frequently and determine if there are *any* potential hazards lurking in the next twenty feet of your path. Pay special attention when you are stepping on to or down from curbs. Don't walk and gaze at your cellphone at the same time, either.

could have caused a "urinary leakage" accident had I not been a younger, sturdier version of my current self.

The solution to Italy's problems would be an army of plaintiff's lawyers like we are so fortunate to have here in the United States (if you're an attorney, that's supposed to be a joke). Although they would instantly sue the hotels into humiliating submission to instigate more safety measures, would it be worth the loss of charm such draconian measures would entail? Many say yes, but I'm not sure.

CHAPTER 2

My Brother-in-Law Steve, the Plumber

I met my future bride shortly after I returned from a year overseas in the Army. Her beauty, kindness, and street-smart savviness swept me off my feet. For the first time in my twenty-nine years, I contemplated marriage. What clinched the deal was when Susie's younger brother Steve commented, "You're so tall!" He grew several inches after that, but there was no going back on the marriage. To be sure, I stood the same five feet, eight inches in one-inch heels as I did when I was known as Legs Gradman in high school.

I started my medical practice several years after we got married, around the same time Steve started his career as a plumber (Fisk-It Plumbing).

He retired—rich and happy, at age fifty-one, about twenty-five years before I retired, burned out and tired at age seventy-six. After that, my respect for tradespeople skyrocketed.

During the course of his career, Steve had occasion to fall-proof many homes. The following is a summary of a discussion we had about the matter.

There are two types of slip and fall accidents—the kind you can sue for and the kind that occur at home. This discussion is limited to the latter.

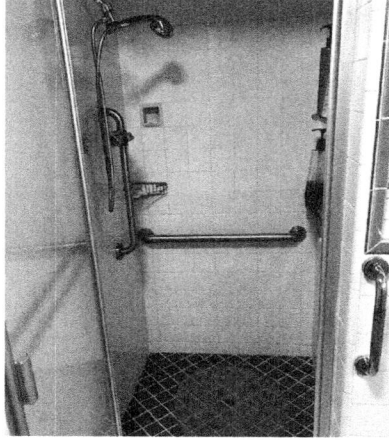

Figure 2. A shower with code-compliant grab bars—two on the inside and one on the outside. Note the circular slip-proof shower pad on the floor.

You must have grab bars in and around all showers and tubs (fig. 2). The walls behind the original tiles can be quite thick, and you can sometimes get away without seeking studs.

Many tub users do not want their back against the faucet, so they face the other way. If so, a *bathtub safety rail* helps to enter and exit the tub (fig. 3).

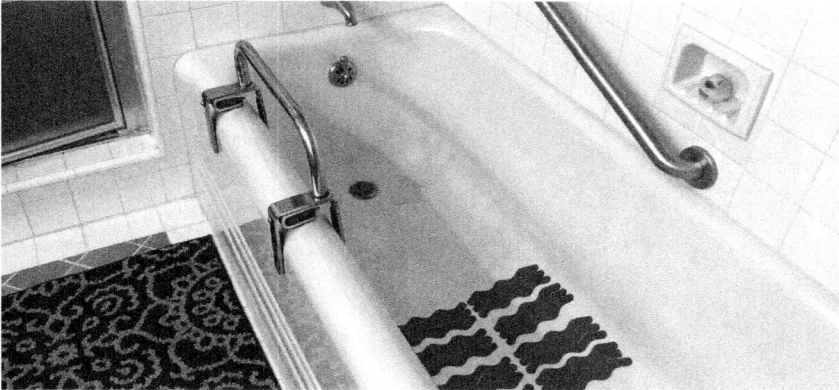

Figure 3. The vertical grab bar adjacent to the tub's faucet and the diagonal grab bar on the wall are required by code. Steve added grab bars when Susie's mom moved into our home. She sat facing the hardware. When Steve learned she disliked getting into and out of the tub at the hardware end, he attached a safety rail on the rim of the tub.

Shower and bath floors are or can become really slippery, especially if the drain stops up. For these reasons you must place a shower mat or apply anti-slip stickers in your shower and tub. Place them wherever you wish. If your tub has a safety rail, place anti-slip stickers kitty corner to it. Furthermore, a mat with a rubberized bottom is preferable to a towel when you exit the shower or tub.

My wife and I recently took a long trip to Europe. We stayed in 3-star, 4-star, and 5-star hotels. Not one of them had the minimum number of grab bars in and around the shower and tub that would meet California code requirements (fig. 4). The shower floors were slippery as well. Susie and I were surprised, disappointed, and frankly concerned for our safety.

Spills are common in kitchens and bathrooms. They should be wiped up immediately. Many commercial kitchens lay rubberized floor mats around their dishwashing stations. These special mats can also be installed in the home. You should install good lighting in the kitchen, not just to prevent slips and falls but for general safety when preparing food.

In the rest of your house, it's better if you *don't* have throw rugs. That's why they call them throw rugs. If you must have one, you should always place an anti-slip mat beneath it. Errant cords can also be problematic.

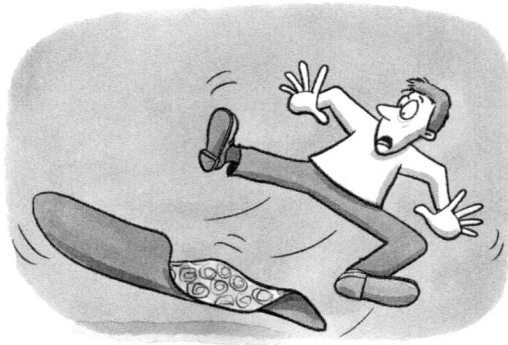

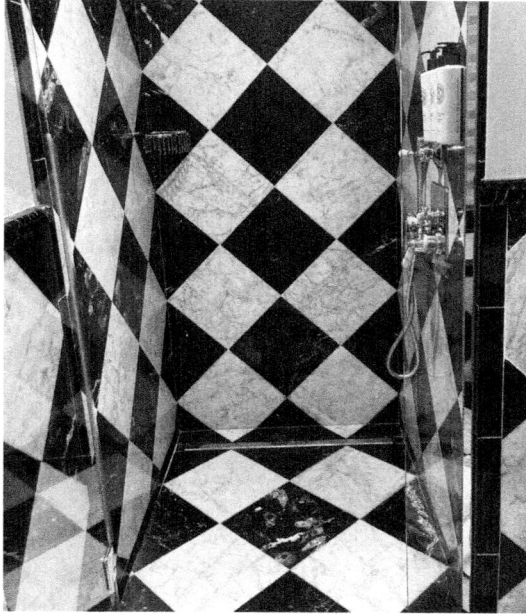

Figure 4. *This shower at a five-star hotel in France has no grab bars inside or outside the shower and no anti-slip stickers or mat on the floor. What could go wrong?*

Both inside and outside the house, the worst flooring is a tie between smooth marble and smooth granite. Water enhances the risk of a serious slip and fall on these slick surfaces (further discussed in chapter 8).

When it comes to using a ladder, the pros know what they're doing, so they seldom have problems. The home repairperson may try to mimic the practiced technique of the professional working across the street, but the amateur has a far higher likelihood of falling off the ladder or, worse, the roof. There is a right way to ascend and descend a ladder and all other ways are wrong.[6]

Another area of great importance are the building codes related to steps. Steps have two parts: the horizontal step itself, called the tread in trade-talk, and the vertical part, which is called the rise. All rises in any given stairway must be of identical height to prevent

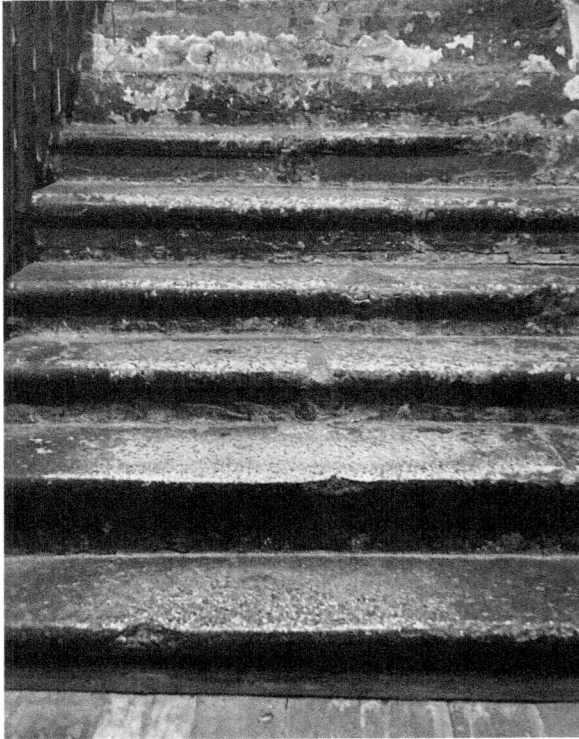

Figure 5. *An old prison with a different rise for each stair.*

erroneously gauging the height between them (fig. 5 is a counter-example).

All outdoor and indoor stairs deserve traction tape. A strip or two of tape is applied to the front of each step, or at least the top and bottom steps, to prevent slippage and visually mark the step as if to signal "This is a step". Outdoor stairs leading to the front door should have the tape completely across the bottom and top stair. The color of the tape should contrast with the underlying material. Non-slip safety strips are available for carpeted stairs as well, but require special installation. If such strips were present in the hotel steps I encountered in Italy, as I described in chapter 1, I suspect I might not have fallen.

MY BROTHER-IN-LAW STEVE, THE PLUMBER

In our family, my wife and I treasure visits to our older son, who blessed us with our first grandchild. I can't begin to tell you how many times we've asked, nay insisted he install low outdoor lights to illuminate the paths and steps that lead from his front door to our parked car on the street. Wouldn't you agree with my wife and me that we should add a clause in our will that leaves him nothing if either my wife or I fall and break a neck when we return to our car at nine o'clock at night?

Strategically placed outdoor lighting is a good idea even if there are no grandparents.

CHAPTER 3

Getting Older

I first noticed I was getting older when police officers and waiters started calling me sir.

Later, I noticed I preferred to sit when I put on pants, socks, and shoes.

It suddenly dawned on me there would come a day when I might need a cane, then a walker, and even a wheelchair if ever I made it into a blue zone—such as Okinawa—where individuals *on average* live over ninety.[7]

After years of caring for her now ninety-eight-year-old mother, my wife realized that staying in our home without the full-time help that her mother would reject anyway, would compromise her safety. So with sad hearts, we placed her at Welbrook Santa Monica, a full-time care facility for individuals with severe memory issues such as Alzheimer's and dementia. The facility itself is spotless, and the staff is enthusiastic, experienced, and competent. She is thriving there.

Although we had encouraged my mother-in-law to use a cane in our home, we weren't sure she really needed it. Welbrook concluded she didn't need one at the time. Two years later she started using a foldup walker to get around.

There is a difference between assisted living facilities, where the decision to use a cane can be left up to the individual, and a memory facility, where the decision often has to be made for the resident.

Many individuals come to Welbrook with the decision already made at home, the hospital, or elsewhere.

The main criterion that determines the day you need an assistive device is when your caregiver sees signs of instability, lack of stamina to walk distances, or you actually fall. The staff at Welbrook encourages more walking rather than less and they prefer your room be further from the dining room rather than closer because of any misguided inclination to save you from too much exertion. Their mantra is "Use it or lose it."

Canes have been around a long time and have been used for more than assistance with walking. They can easily conceal a knife[8] or a small hollowed out portion, perfect for tippling.[9]

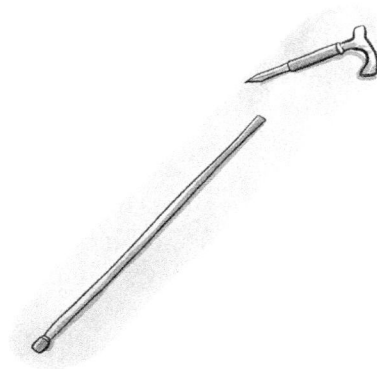

When the word *caning* is used to describe a form of punishment, the reference is not to a wooden cane, but rather to products of rattan palms, the same material used in the tropics to make baskets.

It's helpful to know that some canes can be folded to increase portability. The tip of a cane* should end in a large, flat, rubber attachment to enhance stability and balance. Three- and four-prong canes allow for even more stability and weight-bearing, and are better on stairs. An additional advantage is that the cane will continue to stand

---

 * Otherwise known as a ferrule.

upright when you sit. Further helpful information is discussed on the website mentioned here.[10]

The height of your cane should come roughly up to the bend in your wrist. If your wooden cane is too long, you can cut the bottom end down to the proper height.

If you don't have a bad leg, place the cane in either hand and take your first step with the leg next to the cane. Your next step is with your cane and the other leg.

The first, but unintuitive rule about walking after you have recently had a leg operation or if you have an injured or painful leg, is that you should hold the cane in the hand *on the other side of your good leg*. Take the first step with your good leg. Then swing the cane and bad leg forward. As you move forward, leaning on the cane a little takes weight off the bad leg. This allows you to remain erect and not sway from side to side, thus reducing your chances of falling.

Walking up or down stairs after injury or surgery is more of a challenge. My recommendation—coming, as usual, after considerable personal experience—is to rely on both a cane and a banister. The cane goes in the hand furthest from the banister. When descending stairs, the first move is to lean onto the banister and place the cane on the step below where you are standing. Step down with your bad leg, then follow with your good. If you are ascending the stairs, lean onto the banister and place the cane on the step above. Step up with your good leg, then follow with your bad. A clever way to remember these rules is that the good leg goes to heaven and the bad leg goes to hell. I'll have more to say about ascending and descending a helical stairway in Chapter 6.

Many individuals start using a cane, but possibly for psychological reasons, because they use a cane incorrectly, they fall, or have a fear of falling, quickly conclude they need something with more support, namely a walker. Walkers come in two varieties—the kind you can fold up and throw in the back of your car, and the enhanced variety with brakes, baskets, and real seats. The advantages of the fancy ones are that the brakes are up where your hands are, the basket easily accommodates a purse, and you can sit and rest when you run out of steam. The drawback, of course, is its size and weight, which makes it impractical for transporting. Foldup walkers are more commonly used at Welbrook because they are simple to use, and the staff often takes its residents on outings.

The main rule for using any walker is to step into it and not hunch over to try to push the device from behind.

CHAPTER 4

Oh No! You're Still Recommending Exercise?

The short answer is yes. But allow me another digression. In 1937, Paul Terry became the first person to say, "Whenever I get the urge to exercise, I lie down until the feeling passes." But all he did was tweak some lines from Mark Twain, who wrote, "I have never taken any exercise, except sleeping and resting, and I never intend to take any. Exercise is loathsome."

I know of no greater proponent of that doctrine than my good friend Allen Firstenberg. Although he refused routine exercise, he was a ferocious tennis and basketball player. He died tragically in 2004 of a meningioma at age sixty-two. He was a gentle giant of a guy, with a brain like a rocket scientist—oh wait! He *was* a rocket scientist—Chief of Operations at Rockwell International in Thousand Oaks—but he left that company to start a half billion-dollar software company (in 2003 dollars). He was cut down in the prime of his life and I'm dedicating this chapter to him. He would have loved any set of exercises pared to the absolute minimum.

The challenge is to establish which exercises are essential. How many repetitions are needed? How frequently should you do them? And, what matters most to so many is, what is the least time needed to effect a real difference in fall prevention?

The scientific approach to questions of this nature is first to devise a metric, or test that allows a researcher to quantitate the potential benefit of each exercise regimen. Three of the simplest and most popular are the 10 Meter (25 feet) Walk Test or the near-identical Timed Up and Go (TUG) test, and the 4-Stage Balance Test, all described on the internet. There are many other such tests. Some reflect the needs of the researcher—others, their imagination.

The results of most reported studies show that many exercises can help prevent falls. Although there is good evidence that doing tai chi for an hour every day definitely improves balance,[11] most people don't want to budget that much time for exercise, even for the noble objective of reducing falls.

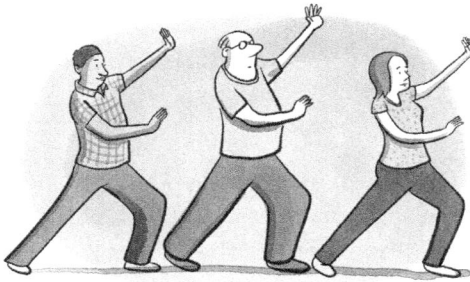

One researcher bravely reported an exercise that *doesn't* help.[12]

None of the reports address the question of what the *minimum* time and effort is needed to reduce the incidence of falls. I believe the law of diminishing returns sets in quickly when it comes to exercises designed to prevent them. Appendix A contains a set of exercises I recommend to improve lower extremity strength, flexibility, and balance. With a little practice, the exercises take roughly ten minutes max and I do them three to four times a week. The benefits of even this minimal regimen greatly outweigh the effort needed to complete them.

Don't confuse these exercises with others designed to maintain good heart health and overall strength. I personally walk four miles at least three times a week while listening to podcasts. While I take these long walks, I often run into Jason Hughes (fig. 6), a passionate exercise guru, whom I lovingly call "the Pushup Nazi", after Larry

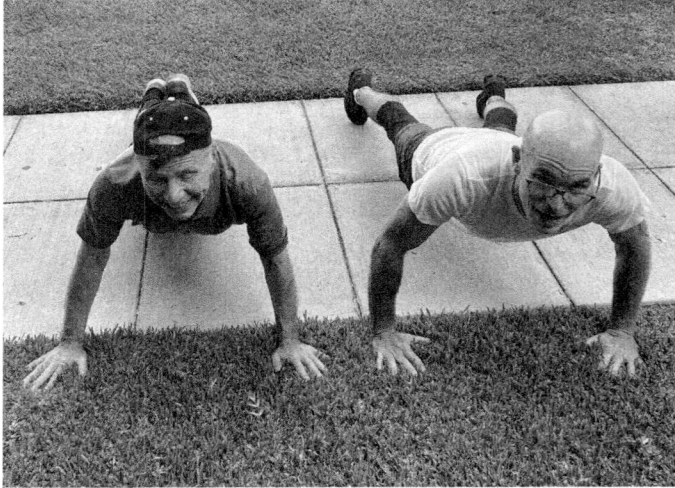

Figure 6. *Jason, the Pushup Nazi and me.*

Thomas, otherwise known as the Soup Nazi on Seinfeld—i.e., someone you love to hate. Jason hangs out just as I turn past the corner onto Roxbury Drive and whenever he's there, he successfully wheedles me into doing 20-25 pushups with him I would otherwise never do. God bless him.

On other days I like to do an hour on a stationary bike while watching fascinating lectures on "The Great Courses Plus", company that produces half hour videos on many fascinating subjects.[13]

CHAPTER 5

Does Weight Play a Role in Falls?

Does obesity (the politically correct word for fat) play a role in the incidence and poor consequences of falls? The short answer is yes.[14] The risk of falls correlates with weights that fall both below normal and in the obese and super obese ranges. The curve resembles a U. People with below normal weight often have bulimia or cancer, **intrinsic** factors (see the Introduction) that are difficult to modify. Not so with people who are overweight.

Successful dieting will lower your body mass index (BMI),* which is, in fact, just a doctor-invented formula that measures the magnitude of your weight taking into consideration your height. Of course your height remains unchanged as you gain or lose weight.† Maintaining a low BMI with weight loss is useful to help prevent falls as long as it doesn't come at the expense of a decrease in muscle mass. The discussion of this tradeoff will become evident when I address the role sarcopenia (muscle wasting) plays in age-associated frailty (see chapter 7).

---

*The word diet used as a noun has two meanings: the first meaning is the food we habitually eat, the second is something you eat for the purpose of losing weight. You should interpret the verb form 'to diet', as used in this chapter, as meaning to eat in such a way as to lose weight.

† If you live a long life, your height will, indeed, become shorter. With aging, you stoop and your spinal discs narrow, thus shortening your overall length. Your height has no bearing on your body mass index (BMI).

One of my insights into the relation between diet and mortality occurred in the early days of my vascular surgery training. My mentor and I were operating on the owner of Shep's Deli, a landmark neighborhood eatery. When we opened his arteries, the cholesterol blocking them oozed out like thick cream.[‡] I had never seen anything like that before, and I've never seen anything like it again. Later, I asked Shep if he ever ate in his delicatessen, and he proudly stated that he ate every single one of his meals there. I promptly instructed Susie never to buy anything at that place again. It closed a few years later.

That story gives me an excuse to tell the pivotal story of how I lost a lot of weight and didn't gain it back. The benefits of that monumental feat remain with me to this day.

To explain: I have a strong family history of coronary artery disease. My father had his first heart attack in his fifties and died at age sixty-nine. He loved all the foods we're discouraged from eating today. He never saw his first grandchild. His horrible history may have nudged me in the direction of my medical specialty. Here I was, a vascular surgeon who should have known better, racking up the pounds because for some unknown reason I chose one of the most stressful specialties in medicine. My father and I were addicted to what I lovingly call *my* version of the four main food groups—bread, pasta, rice, and potatoes. When I finally tipped the scale at 185, I realized I had to change my eating habits.

I turned to my eldest son, who had recently lost weight, for advice. His answer was the paleo diet (from the Greek word *palaiós*, meaning old or ancient).

For a scientist like me, that simple recommendation raised obvious questions. What did our hunter-gatherer ancestors actually eat? Given that hunter-gatherers were probably not losing weight every day, why would duplicating what they ate result in weight loss? Doesn't exercise play a role, too?

[‡] The cholesterol buildup that usually blocks arteries (hardening of the arteries) has the consistency of a pencil's eraser. Remember those?

The answers to these questions are more complex than they sound. Herman Pontzer, PhD, a professor of evolution anthropology at Duke University, authored a captivating book about the history of humans, the hunter-gatherer (i.e., paleo) diet, exercise, and related topics.[15]

The following discussion is my attempt to apply his knowledge and research findings to the issue of whether the paleo diet was the answer to my little "weight issue".

The ancestors that gave rise to today's Homo sapiens appeared about two million years ago as a new species called Homo erectus. They were among the first members of the new genus, Homo.[§]

Several traits appearing in the Homo genus made them unique. These include using stone tools, having a brain larger than their primate ancestors, foraging and hunting for their food, and eventually using fire to cook it. To this long and impressive list, Dr. Pontzer adds the socially useful custom of sharing food.

Anthropologists attend endless meetings that address the precise timing of the astonishing behavioral and physical changes in humans around two million years ago, give or take a million. But from where this amateur sits, an awful lot of very important changes were introduced at roughly the same time. Putting them in definitive chronological order will be a daunting task for future anthropology PhD candidates.

Offshoots of Homo erectus include Homo neanderthalensis (the Neanderthals), who branched off about 300,000 years ago but mysteriously fizzled out about 40,000 years ago, Homo denisova (the Denisovans), who lived on the Tibetan Plateau, and Homo sapiens, the species that dominates our world today. Even though all the

---

[§]How can you remember what these designations mean? Most mnemonics biologists and doctors use are pornographic (Ask one!) A sanitized version of taxonomy (a way to classify plants and animals based on shared characteristics) is King Philip Came for Good Soup. We humans are in the Kingdom Animalia, the Phylum Cordate, the Class Mammal, the Genus Homo, and the Species Homo sapiens, the only species of the Homo genus still around today. Homo erectus, the Neanderthals and the Denisovans died out thousands of years ago.

other species of Homo have died out, we Homo sapiens still have bona fide hunter-gatherer societies scattered around the world today that give us important insights into the diet of our pre-historic ancestors.

The Homo diet that hunter-gatherers ate (and continue to eat today), includes lean meat, fish, fruits, honey, nuts, seeds, vegetables, some natural whole wheat grains, and large quantities of tubers.

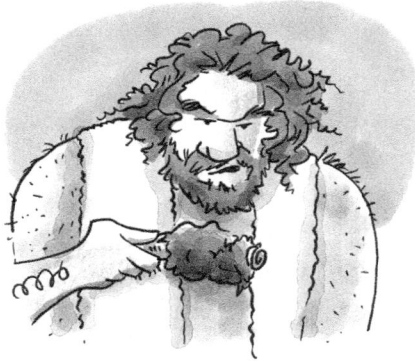

Tubers are specialized parts of an underground plant stem with buds that allow for plant reproduction. They contain starchy complex carbohydrates.¶ Potatoes and yams are examples of tubers, but the large potatoes and yams we eat today are a product of intense cultivation. Hunter-gathers also scavenge for honey and fruit—both high in simple glucose—along with other vegetables.

What hunter-gatherers do *not* eat are refined carbohydrates, dairy, legumes, or anything that typically tumbles out of a vending machine.** Most of the bread, pasta, and rice we consume today has been refined and contain much less nutritional value than what nature provides.

¶A complex carbohydrate contains simple sugars that are woven together into a much larger molecule, which slows their breakdown into simple sugars in the body.

**Refined carbohydrates refer to milled grains that have their outer bran removed, thus stripping the grain of its fiber and antioxidants.

Hunter-gatherers then and today mostly hunt animals with little fat, so by default, their paleo diet differs from today's keto diet, which resembles the paleo diet, but allows eating the fat and marbled meat found in domesticated animals.

Despite having no access to refined carbohydrates, past hunter-gatherer societies consumed most of their calories in the form of carbohydrates, as do hunter-gatherer societies today. The hunter-gatherer diet is by no means low in calories, and with the exception of dairy products, refined carbohydrates, and legumes, is the same as ours.

Dr. Pontzer intensively studies the Hadza people who live in Tanzania. They have maintained a traditional foraging lifestyle that is about as close to that of our hunter-gatherer ancestors as a researcher could hope.

Dr. Pontzer noted that Hadza men spend long hours every day hunting for animals both large and small. Women, likewise, spend many hours seeking and digging tubers from the ground. Thus, the Hadza people expend prodigious calories just trying to fill their bellies. You would be excused if you concluded that the *total* calories they expend every day should equal the prodigious calories they expend while walking on the trails or digging for tubers, plus the baseline calories they expend while doing nothing, like when they sleep or eat.[††]

You would, however, be wrong.

Dr. Pontzer was able to calculate the total calories individuals burn daily with the help of an elegant chemical test that uses isotopes. He noted that there is a slight bump in total calories with normal activities, but nothing earthshaking. But he really did expect to see a large increase in the calorie expenditure of Hazda men, who walk from sunup to sundown every day. He was surprised to learn that the Hadza men consume and burn off roughly 2600 calories every

[††]The basal metabolic rate is the number of calories consumed at rest. This averages 1700 calories a day for a typical man and 1550 calories for a woman. This is more than half the calories you consume daily.

day,[‡‡] little more than any well-fed adult in the world today. Other researchers have confirmed Dr. Pontzer's findings.

Does Dr. Pontzer conclude that strenuous exercise or work does *not* require the Hadza to consume a proportionately larger number of calories every day? The glaringly counterintuitive answer is yes! That's a mega bummer if you and every personal trainer and exercise studio in the world would have you believe that vigorous exercise alone will slim you down and give you the body of your dreams.

Dr. Pontzer explains this enigmatic finding by noting that

> the body makes room for the [energy] cost of additional activity by reducing the calories spent on the many unseen tasks that take up most of our daily energy budget [our basal metabolic rate]—the housekeeping work that our cells and organs do to keep us alive.[16] Saving energy on these processes could make room in our daily energy budget, allowing us to spend more on physical activity without increasing total calories spent per day. For example, exercise often reduces inflammatory activity that the immune system mounts, as well as levels of reproductive hormones such as estrogen[17] . . . All of this evidence points toward obesity being a disease of gluttony rather than sloth.

In other words, we humans are programmed to burn the same number of calories every day, so if you use more than the customary amount to exercise, your organs and cells will cut back on their basal metabolic rate so that, in the end, the total calories you consume and burn off daily remains the same.

If true, it means that **there is no escaping the need for you to reduce calorie intake** if you ever expect to lose weight.

[‡‡] Of course, there are outliers. Olympic swimmer Michael Phelps, who won eight gold medals in Beijing in 2008 and a career total of twenty-three gold medals, self-reported that he routinely ate 12,000 calories each day for years while training. His diet was high in fatty meats, refined carbohydrates, and saturated fats in bulk, but he somehow burned off all those "unhealthy" calories and remained thin.

DOES WEIGHT PLAY A ROLE IN FALLS?

I didn't know all this when I long ago asked myself what I should do about my weight. My career choice didn't allow me to add much exercise to my 24-7 vascular practice anyway. So, I would have to rely on a low-calorie diet. I was shaky on the paleo diet, only because I wasn't sure what it was and how it worked. In the end, I chose to completely eliminate my beloved "four main food groups", even though doing so doesn't duplicate the true paleo diet, which restricts dairy but allows complex carbohydrates in the form of tubers like potatoes. For breakfast, I substituted nuts for cereal, added abundant berries (non-refined carbs), and a little yogurt for its calcium.

Unknowingly, I was complying with the *sine qua non* for losing weight—i.e., reducing calorie intake, especially refined carbohydrates. For me, the diet was surprisingly easy to maintain. I was delighted when the pounds melted away. I got down to about 150 pounds and happily filled my closet with new clothes.

I pretty much stick to this diet today. After going off his "paleo" diet, my son regrettably regained his original weight. After a little nagging, he decided to go on low carbohydrate diet similar to mine. His diet avoids the same refined carbohydrates as the paleo diet, but permits fatter meats (the keto diet). He supplements that with lots of exercise. He's already lost thirty pounds and he looks and feels great.

I, too, looked and felt better, my blood pressure and cholesterol levels dropped, and I slept better. Because I don't waddle anymore, I am confident my risk of falling has dropped.

So shouldn't I recommend a low carb diet to everyone? Well, hold your horses. A recent review of diets concludes that diets "that are very low or low in carbohydrates result in weight loss that equivalent to—not better than—that achieved with other diets that have a higher carbohydrate content."[18] That was something I was not expecting to read. The only conclusion that appears to be universally true in the world of dieting is a related study that shows that the most crucial factor in maintaining weight loss is **adherence** to the weight-loss diet of your choice, not the specific diet.[19]

The recent introduction of weight-loss drugs—originally crafted for diabetics—may be a huge gift to the obese. Recent studies show they are relatively safe and effective even if you don't have diabetes.[20] If time shows there are latent side-effects of these drugs, or if the price of the drugs remain prohibitive, you could and should revert to a calorie-limiting diet.

I would love to say the frequency of my falls decreased after I lost all that weight. For a while, though, my falls, continued apace.[§§] Researching this book is what finally *did* put an end to my own falls.

————— SELECT YOUR DIET AND STICK TO IT —————

The most important factor in maintaining weight loss if you are overweight is **adherence** to the reduced calorie diet of your choice, not the specific diet.

[§§]That observation does not negate the fact that weight-loss reduces the incidence of falls.

CHAPTER 6

Stairs and Banisters

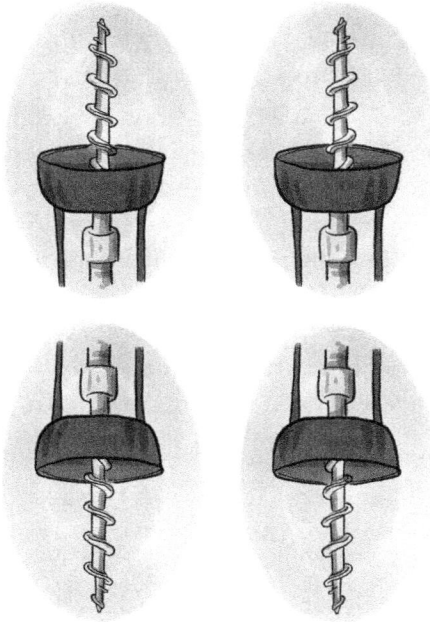

The top and bottom cork-screws on the left are both left-handed and clockwise.

The top and bottom cork-screws on the right are both right-handed and counter-clockwise.

hapter 1 was concerned mostly with falls on a flat surface. If you fall upward while ascending stairs, your injury is typically low impact and doesn't often result in broken bones. On the other hand, falls on descending stairs occur more frequently.[21] Furthermore, you are subject to significantly greater injury on impact, which increases the further you fall. In a study of 118 patients who fell down stairs and entered the emergency room with suspected multiple injuries, 80% suffered a traumatic brain injury, often fatal.[22] It follows you should be extra careful going down stairs.

My uncle Sam was about as healthy a hundred-year-old as you'll ever meet. He ate apples for breakfast, was still successfully investing in the stock market (well, better than I ever did, but that's a low bar), and *ran* twice daily with his beloved frisky schnauzer Peppy until he was ninety-five. His house was multilevel, with five to six wide steps between floors. One day, while descending one set of these stairs, he pitched forward while not holding on to the banister. A CT scan showed a fractured skull and a large cerebral bleed. Although he lived a few more years, none were productive.

My father-in-law David Fiske lived to age ninety-five. He too was reasonably healthy until the very end. A couple of years before he passed, he visited a neighbor and encountered a recently built helical stairway that had a wall with no banister on the outside curve, and no wall or banister on the inside curve. I am confident the stairway was not up to the then-current building codes. He tried to take care descending, but he fell and broke several ribs. Is there some way he could have prevented that fall? Yes. He could have sat on the top step and bumped his way down. But without having thought about it beforehand, my father-in-law did not "stumble" upon the solution. Or if he had, being the curmudgeonly but loveable soul he was, he defiantly tried to descend the stairs upright anyway.

The space-saving footprint and aesthetic charm of helical stairways (one shaped like a corkscrew) are two reasons homeowners and builders favor them for two-story homes. They preserve space, but allow only one person to go up or down at a time easily. Helical stairways are inherently far more dangerous than straight staircases

---

DESCENDING STAIRS

As you age, it becomes increasingly important to use a banister when descending stairs.

because they usually have only one banister, on the inside curve, and have a narrower tread there as well. For these reasons I will spend more time discussing them.

As you age, you will increasingly use a banister to descend stairs. It is better to rely on a banister rather than a cane when you descend stairs because banisters don't wobble.

Helices are a fascinating object of study. Organisms shaped like a helix are common in nature. My grandson Dash has a next-door neighbor named Helix and they are the best of friends. Helix is thin, but he's not shaped like a helix. Helicobacter pylori, the bacterium responsible for stomach ulcers and some cancers, is not only shaped like a helix, but also swims in a helix-like pattern. I wouldn't be surprised if the organism is shaped like a helix to preserve space, and swims in a helix-like pattern to make swimming more efficient. If this is true, it might be the first example wherein nature follows stairway design.

Helices come in two distinct forms. The relation between them is like your right and left hands—they are mirror images of each other, but cannot be superimposed.

Furthermore, each of the two helical forms can be described in two ways—as being either (1) right-handed or left-handed, or (2) curving clockwise or counterclockwise. This dual property, known as **chirality,** * is important in many branches of biology and science, not just staircases. If a staircase, or any other helix is right-handed, it is also counterclockwise. If it is left-handed, it is clockwise.

----

*Pronounced with a hard k

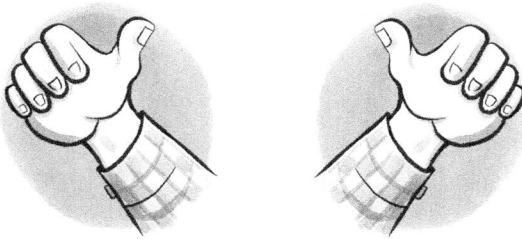

The handedness of a helix appears the same when you look down at it from the other end. This property can be hard to appreciate, but the figures heading this chapter can help you understand why this is true.

The DNA of all living organisms consists of two intertwined helices, each of which is right-handed.

Almost all manufactured screws, corkscrews, and jars with tops are right-handed, i.e., by turning them with your right hand, the screw moves forward either into the wall, into the cork, or tightens the jar onto its top. This is the practical definition of whether a helix is right-handed or left-handed. It also gives rise to the handyman's mnemonic, "righty tighty, lefty loosey".

Helical staircases, which are about half the staircases used in two-story homes, on the other hand, are defined from the point of view of a person standing at the bottom of the staircase looking up. The staircase in our home (fig. 7) is both right-handed and counter-clockwise.

Straight staircases usually come with two banisters, one on either side of the steps. Our staircase originally came with a banister only on the inside curve, which is typical of helical stairways built before stricter building codes advised otherwise. If you have nothing in either hand, you could use the inside banister to assist with your descent, but you are then obliged to use narrower steps than you should. Your situation was worse if you had, say, a coffee cup in your right hand. You could no longer use the banister and you were descending the stairs with nothing to grab onto if you stumbled. Of course, you could have switched hands before descending, but for most of us it's too much of a bother. As usual, I'm in the "most of us" category. Thus, helical stairways pose a far greater fall hazard than a straight one.

Today, the International Building Code still requires only one banister for new residential helical stairways. California, the bluest of blue states, recommends two,[23] but as Hamlet says in the eponymous play, "More honor'd in the breach than the observance."

STAIRS AND BANISTERS

My ever-vigilant wife saw an accident just waiting to happen. Ms. Prophylaxis hired an ironmonger to build a second banister on the outer curve of the stairway. Ironmongers usually hang out at hardware stores. If you can't find one, just have someone build it out of wood. Either way, it's a custom job but the risk-benefit ratio greatly favors having a second banister. Now that the second banister is in place, I reflexively place my left hand on the outside banister to descend whether I'm carrying a coffee cup in my right hand or not.

The benefit of having two banisters on any stairway is not limited to those occasions when you carry a coffee cup downstairs. At some time during your life, you may find yourself in a situation in which you are obliged to bear more weight on your right leg than the left.[†] Examples include following surgery on your left foot for a neuroma or back pain relieved by putting more weight on your right leg. These examples are common, and we are grateful that the second banister was in place before our time of need, when installing one would have been too late.

Chairlifts and elevators also have their place when contemplating the potential hazards of staircases, but they are relatively expensive.

High impact falls are not just limited to stairs. I once found a random newspaper lying on an elevated area of our lawn. As I advanced to it from uphill, I reached over and nearly toppled down the hill. But with my newly acquired flexibility skills (appendix A), I deftly escaped a major tumble. Had I encountered this situation after I drafted this book, I would have known to pick up the newspaper by approaching the newspaper from downhill. If I fell, it would have been uphill, not downhill.

Helical stairs are often a feature of medieval castle towers. They were the key point of entry to the living quarters of the rulers and their defense was crucial in deciding if the invaders or the defendants prevailed when outsiders attacked a castle. This topic arises any time a tour guide enters a castle that has a helical staircase.

[†] I'm using our home's counterclockwise stairway as an example.

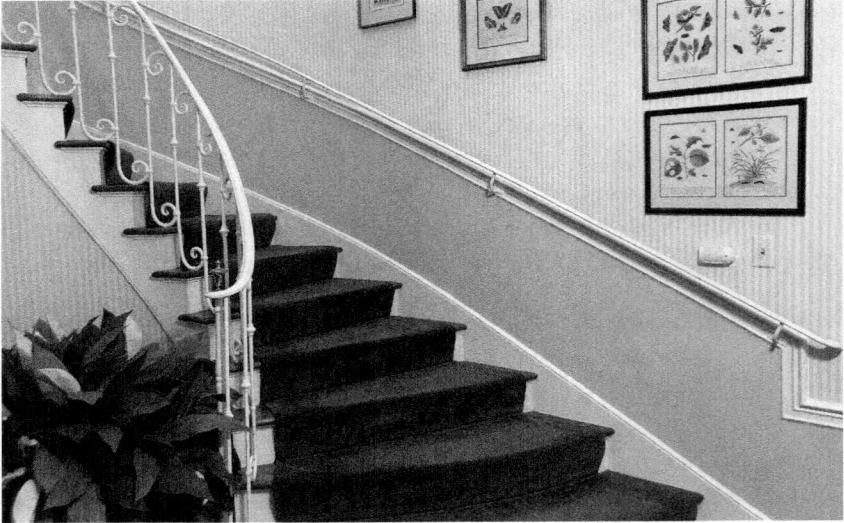

Figure 7. *This is the helical stairway in our home. It runs right-handed and counter-clockwise. We installed the iron banister on the wall.*

Guides are fond of explaining that in mediaeval times, the castle defender, who in battle would normally stand higher on the staircase because he was defending the castle, always constructed his tower staircase with whichever configuration would allow him to have more freedom to slash at the intruder and push him down the stairs. Most of the "experts" who wade into this issue argue that clockwise staircases favor the defender standing higher on the staircase, but there are many stubborn nay-sayers who question that belief.

─────────── **BANISTERS ON HELICAL STAIRCASES** ───────────

If your home has a helical staircase, construct a second banister on the outside wall.

This is a surprisingly hot button issue and I have my own take on the matter. My guide in Lithuania, Iga, is the assailant and she is attacking while ascending a left-handed clockwise staircase (fig. 8). If she wants more room to slash the castle's defender (presumably me), she will instinctively move to her left, where the stairs are wider—better for her. Conversely, if I want more room to use my right hand, I will need to move to my left, where the stairs are much narrower and thus more hazardous. Thus, it is the assailant who would appear to have the advantage climbing a clockwise staircase.[24]

But, I believe that the more critical issue in battles that took place on helical staircases is that whoever stood higher on the staircase was in a more favorable position to *decapitate* the enemy, while the assailant was more likely to injure only the defender's legs.

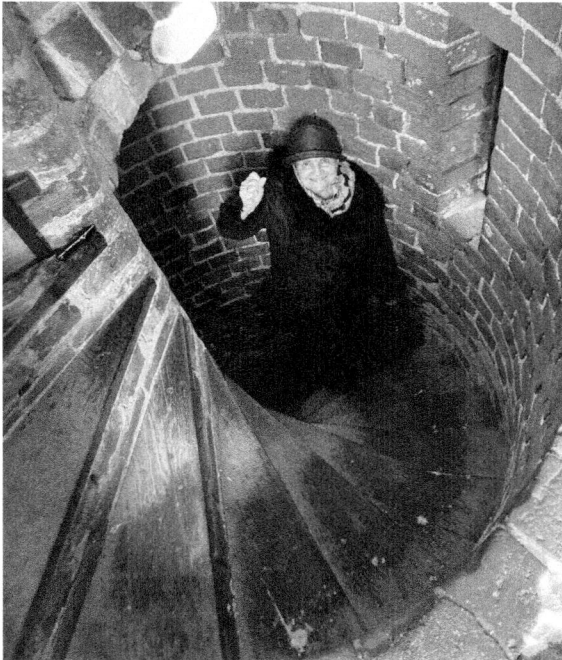

Figure 8. *Off with her head! My guide Iga brandishes her imaginary sword ready to hack my knees. I, on the other hand, defending from above and looking down the stairs, find her head to be the more tempting target. From both my point of view and Iga's, the staircase appears left-handed and clockwise. Note that each step narrows almost to nothing adjacent to the center of the helix. This photo was taken in a fourteenth century Lithuanian tower.*

For that reason, I do not think medieval tower staircase designers gave the chirality (handedness) of the staircase much thought in the first place.

Medieval castle staircase design speculators also argue that the non-uniform treads and rises of some castle staircase steps were intentional.[25] These are known today as "stumble steps". This theory argues that an intruder unfamiliar with the stairs will stumble on them, whereas the defenders would be aware of the variations and would hold their footing. I disagree here as well. This argument makes no sense if you consider that the "preferred" clockwise configuration of the staircase leads the tower defender to move instinctively to the inner part of each step, where intimate knowledge of the pattern of stair rise is unlikely. I suspect stumble steps resulted solely from poor construction, not anticipation of invasion. There are simply too many medieval staircases with a uniform stair rise (such as the pictured castle staircase).

CHAPTER 7

"Frailty, thy Name is Woman"

Shakespeare was fifty-two when he died, but that age was much older than the average life expectancy of his time, which was only twenty-five.* Today, with more centenarians surviving each year, we more commonly use the word frailty in its physical sense.† An outstanding review of frailty in older adults may be found in the endnotes.[26]

Shakespeare knew nothing about sarcopenia and telomere shortening, two important concepts that characterize aging. They were discovered and characterized within the past one hundred years.

The word *sarcopenia*, which literally translates to *muscle wasting*, says it all. Sarcopenia is a major cause of frailty in the aged, along with chronic inflammation and mutations in the body's mitochondria (the tiny parts of every cell that make the energy each cell needs to survive.) Furthermore, when you modify your diet to lose weight, you might actually lose muscle mass along with the fat.[27] Your body doesn't always distinguish between the two.

---

*Childhood deaths were much more common then, due to the very high toll of infectious diseases in the young. Today, vaccines and antibiotics effectively eliminate most serious childhood infections that were so common until the twentieth century.

†Shakespeare, of course, was not referring to the frailty of women as they age, although women do live longer than men and have a higher incidence of osteoporosis that make them more prone to bone fractures if they fall. Shakespeare was referring to the spiritual frailty of Hamlet's mother, Gertrude, who remarried so quickly after her husband died.

Sarcopenia is the subject of intense medical research today. What we do know is that you can slow but not eliminate the advance of sarcopenia with resistance and weight training exercises. That is another reason why exercise is an important adjunct to overall health whether or not you are dieting. Sarcopenia, along with its consequent frailty, is a major contributor to falls.

I recently met a woman who told me her parents frequently fall. She observed that both had become frail. I told her they must start using a cane and she thanked me for the advice. I heard the same story from my financial adviser the next day. If you have elderly parents who are frail and at risk of falling, you must step in and advocate strenuously (often over vigorous objections) for simple measures, such as using a banister and a cane, that could avert a catastrophic life-changing accident.

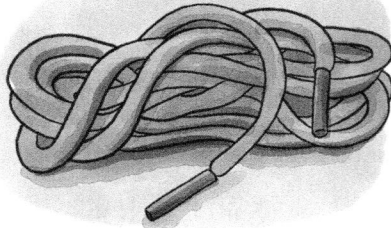

Hermann Muller, a German botanist, discovered telomeres in 1938. Telomeres are special structures found at both ends of all chromosomes in both animals and plants. Humans have forty-six chromosomes. Each time a cell divides, a small amount of DNA is lost from each telomere end. I like the analogy between ageing telomeres and the aglets (tips) of a shoelace.

When you run out of telomeres, you run out of life. Regrettably, telomere shortening implies there is a theoretical upper limit to the human life span, estimated to be 150 years.

To be sure, researchers are furiously seeking a solution to this limitation, and some are pinning their hopes on CRISPR/Cas9 technology, which is a means of inserting genes directly into the DNA of almost all organisms, including humans. That could one day include lengthening telomeres. This pioneering technology was developed by Jennifer Doudna, PhD, for which she justifiably received the Nobel Prize for Chemistry in 2020. The technique is already being used to treat hemophilia. Another way to extend telomere life would be to find a medication that disables the enzyme that shortens telomeres.

Wouldn't you sign up for an injection that could keep telomeres from disappearing, thus conferring additional years of functioning life?

CHAPTER 8

The Treachery of Ice and Other Slippery Surfaces

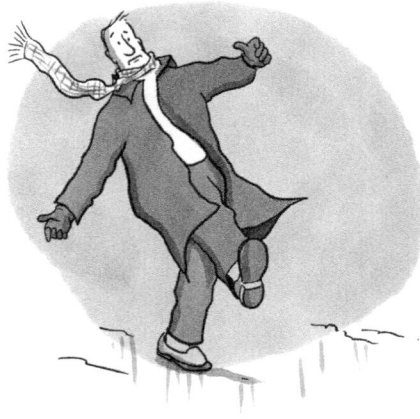

Following a recent flight, our plane parked about fifty yards from the ground floor entrance to the terminal. All of us had to walk the short distance hauling whatever carry-on luggage we brought on board. The temperature hovered around freezing, and a drizzle of icy rain covered the ground.

The first man off the plane was dressed in a business suit, large over-coat, and smooth soled dress shoes. He took three confident steps and promptly fell onto the tarmac.

The word *tarmac* is a portmanteau, meaning it combines two words—in this case tar and macadam. Macadam, named after its inventor,

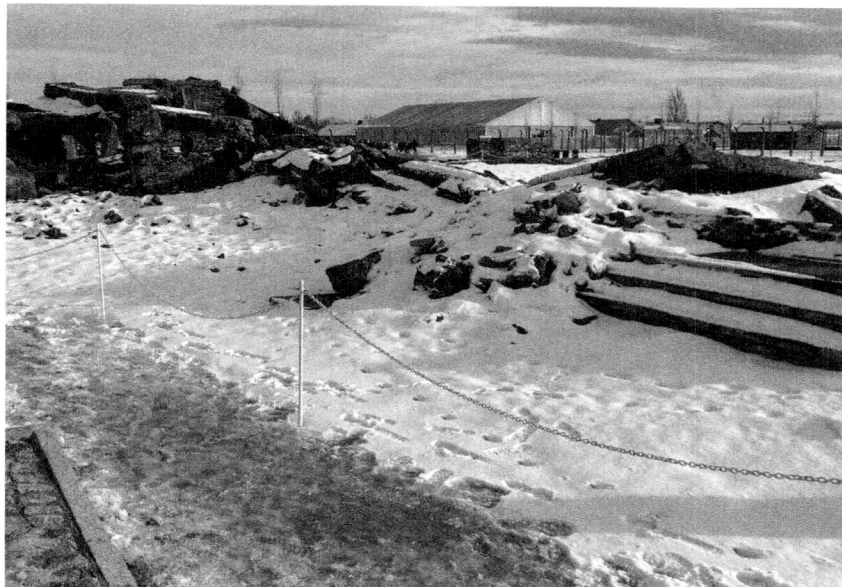

Figure 9. A patch of slippery black ice menaces in the foreground. It was far easier to walk in the snow.

John McAdam, is just another word for asphalt. When aviation personnel use the word tarmac, they also include the runways, which are made of cement, not asphalt.

His bulky overcoat reduced the chances of a fracture. After he brushed himself off, the gentleman instinctively started taking baby steps and successfully made it to the terminal.

There are lessons here for all, but first a little background. Our remote hominids walked on all fours, leaving their body's center of gravity shared among four legs. Falling is rare in four-legged animals. About five million years ago, pre- humans (like gorillas and chimpanzees) started walking on two legs, leaving both hands free to do more important things. This major leap forward came at a price, namely the possibility of losing balance and falling at any time. Walking has often been described as controlled falling. Evolution, however, has adapted the human nervous system to select the best spot to place our feet and stabilize our center of gravity with each step. Rarely does an adult lose his balance and fall for this reason.[28]

Since the tarmac was black and the icy covering thin and thus transparent, the condition we encountered is called "black ice". Black ice may appear to be safe, but it is exceedingly slippery (fig. 9). Walking on a slippery surface like ice or sleety rain greatly increases the likelihood of falling. In the US, a million people fall on ice every year, of which 17,000 are fatal.[29]

So what do you do if you find yourself surrounded by ice? Some of you may question my bona fides for discussing this matter since I live in California, but I assure you that I survived many a windy Chicago winter in early global warming days, when temperatures often dropped below zero degrees Fahrenheit and ice was everywhere.

All ice over about -5C° (t 23°F) and under 0C° (32° F, the melting point of ice) is naturally covered by an exceedingly thin layer of water. Within **microseconds** of standing or walking on that ice, or scraping over it with skates or a sled, the very thin layer of water increases to a somewhat thicker layer of water. With the added water, the slightly melted ice becomes very slippery.

Leonardo DaVinci was the first to describe the basic properties of friction. He understood there was a relation between the roughness of an object and its resistance to slipping.

To understand anything about friction, you need to know about the coefficient of friction (often abbreviated as COF or with the Greek letter μ.) The COF measures the amount of friction between two surfaces, and runs between 0.0 (the most slippery possible) and 1.0 (the least slippery possible). Table 1 gives the coefficient of friction for some common surface pairs.

Rubber on wet concrete has the same slipperiness as rubber on wood and the COF is sufficiently high μ = 0.70), so if you are wearing rubber soled shoes, you will rarely fall on either.

Appendix B is a somewhat more thorough and mathematically oriented explanation of friction. It is optional and should be avoided by those who are math-phobic.

THE TREACHERY OF ICE AND OTHER SLIPPERY SURFACES

TABLE 1

	μ	
Ice on ice	0.10	[Notice how slippery ice is]
Steel on ice	0.14	Ice skating
Rubber on ice	0.15	Walking on ice with rubber soled shoes
Leather on wood	0.35	Walking on wood with leather soled shoes
Rubber on wet concrete	0.70	Walking outside on a rainy day
Rubber on wood	0.70	Walking on wood with rubber shoes
Rubber on dry concrete	0.90	Walking on the side walk with rubber shoes

I offer five recommendations to avoid falling on slippery surfaces:

The **first** is to grab a handrail if one is available. Even with a handrail, however, descending icy stairs is a scary task. Walking in *uncompacted* snow next to the stairs is less dangerous than walking on ice so if there is uncompacted snow next to the stairs, use it to walk your way down. Another option is to sit on the top stair and inch your way down step by step, holding the banister if you can. Inelegant, but it gets the job done.

The **second** is to take baby steps or, as some prefer, penguin steps, since babies fall and penguins seldom do. Penguins and other animals that don't fall on ice are discussed further at the end of this chapter, and penguin steps are also discussed in Addendum B.

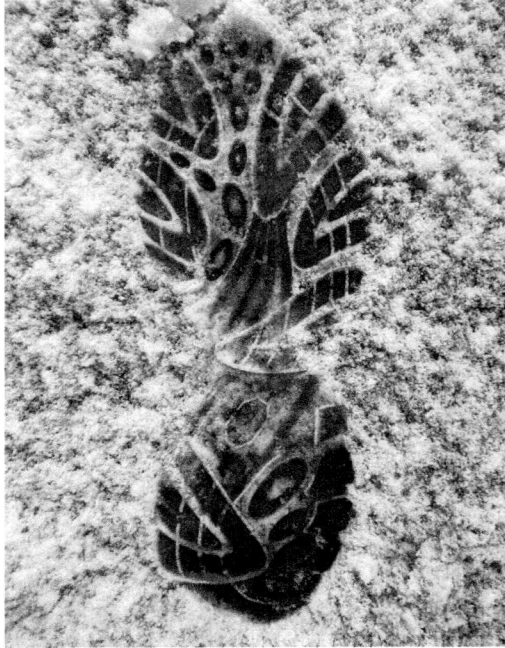

Figure 10. *My shoe tread has grooves both large and small that squeezes water out when I take a step.*

The **third** is to focus on the slip/fall resistant properties of the shoes themselves. There are two ways to approach this issue. The first is to improve the slip resistant properties of the shoe material itself.

Rubber, which is already slip resistant on dry surfaces like wood and concrete, is used in 30% of shoe-soles world-wide. It is durable, frost resistant, and inexpensive. Replacement candidates for walking on ice include soles made of thermoplastic rubber, polyvinyl chloride, polyurethane, thermoplastic polyurethane, thermoplastic elastomers, ethylene vinyl acetate, and others. The manufacturers of Vibram Arctic grip shoes and boots have gritty fiberglass fillers embedded into their soles that allow hikers to walk up icy slopes as steep as 7%.

A related approach to avoiding slips and falls on ice is to use shoes or boots with either large-scale or small-scale treads. Contrary to first impressions, a pattern with ridges facing in all directions (fig. 10) is not necessarily better than a pattern that is more regular. One major goal in wearing treaded shoes is for the water that accumulates in the spaces between the treads to run off the sides when you take a step, because your weight squeezes some of the water out. Decreasing the amount of water in contact with the bottom of your shoe increases the effective static COF and makes walking safer.

The **fourth** recommendation involves increasing traction with hiking poles or shoe enhancements.[30] Many years ago, Finnish hikers began to use paired hiking poles to enhance upper body fitness while walking or trekking over difficult terrain. Today this is known as Nordic hiking. These same poles provide balance and stability when walking on icy city streets. The tungsten carbide tips that come with the poles easily grip ice, thus improving traction. To walk at home on more delicate surfaces like wood, just place ferrules over the tungsten carbide tips (figs. 11 and 12).

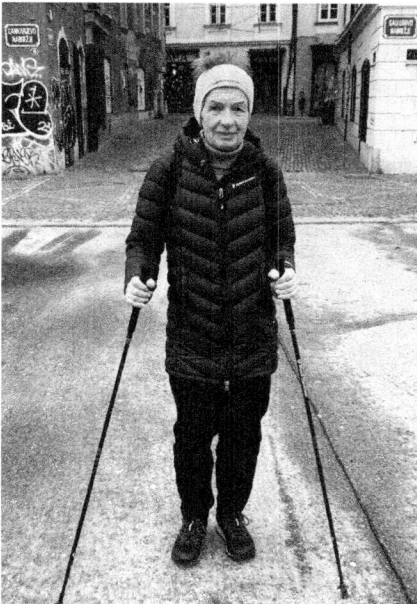

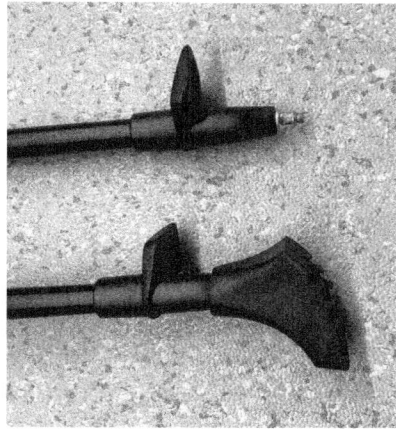

Figure 12. The top pole has a tungsten carbide tip. The bottom pole has an attached rubber bootie for walking indoors.

Figure 11. Walking with poles in icy conditions.

Ice cleats take this concept one step further with sharp multipronged ice grabbers easily attached around or to the bottom of your shoes. Good choices for city walking are the Yaktrax ICEtrekkers Diamond Grip Traction Device and EXOspikes.* If you need or want to climb icy mountains, you'll need crampons, which have multiple spikes emerging from a plate firmly attached to the bottom of your boot.

Together, a combination of common sense, baby steps, and special shoes and devices should keep you out of trouble if you anticipate walking in an icy situation. We humans didn't evolve to thrive surrounded by ice (an observation that weighed heavily in my decision to emigrate from Chicago to Los Angeles).

How do some members of the animal kingdom manage to live, forage, and reproduce in harsh winters.[31]

Polar bears walk on their forefeet, and, like, humans, also walk on their heels. Their paw pads are exceptionally large to begin with, but with each step, the bear's massive weight spreads the pads out even more, which squeezes the water out of the spaces between their paw pads and the ice. Both actions increase the effective COF of their paws. In addition, their forefeet and hindfeet also have many prominent spike-like structures called papillae that add considerable gritty traction to their gait. Finally, polar bears have sharp non-retractable claws that they use to initiate walking and assist in moving forward and climbing. This multicombination approach gives polar bears extraordinary traction on ice. Polar bears can travel hundreds of miles at a fast clip and not fall.

Seals spend about half their time in the water seeking food. They emerge onto land to rest, play, give birth, and molt. Even though seals appear to have no hair, they all have growing fur. Seals thus need to molt periodically, which keeps them sleek in the water—like getting a new Speedo every year. Compared to their swiftness in water, seals typically lumber slowly on ice. They have sharp claws on their front flippers that can grasp the ice and assist with forward motion,

---

*Trey French. "The Best Ice Cleats for Shoes," *New York Times*, December 14, 2023.

but they can also advance using their stomach muscles alone. On video, it appears that their muscles are sequentially undulating up and down like a caterpillar does when moving forward.[32] When seals move very quickly, they actually look like they are bouncing forward. Their short belly fur gets very stiff when wet and penetrates the ice, thus augmenting forward movement.

A close look at the paw pads of polar bears and seals shows abundant long hair curled to fill the spaces between the gripping surfaces. This hair may be useful for insulation, but it may also serve as a reservoir of water that gets squeezed out when the animal steps on each foot. The effect is to dry the hair out and increase the effective COF.

Humans do not grow hair on their feet and soles. The evolutionary rationale could be that humans need hair-free hands to grip tools, but the actual genetic reason remained a mystery until University of Pennsylvania researchers discovered that humans have a protein inhibitor, Dickkopf 2 (DKK2), that suppresses hair follicles from growing hair on both palms and soles.[33]

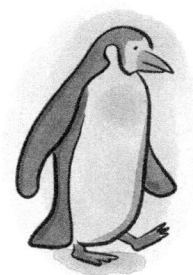

Penguins are flightless birds but, like seals, accomplished swimmers. They have a relatively low center of gravity except when they get fat gorging on fish. To avoid toppling, fat penguins must move slowly and deliberately.[†] Penguins use their clawed feet to grasp ice, and like the polar bear, their footpad and webbed feet are divided into

---

[†] Compare this with the same issue humans face, which I discussed early in this chapter.

TOSCANINI'S SHOES

The risk of falling on a slippery surface confronted Arturo Toscanini (1867-1957), who conducted the New York Philharmonic Orchestra from 1928 to 1936. I agree with many critics who proclaim Toscanini to be the twentieth century's finest conductor. He was well known for his passionate conducting style. His arms flailed in all directions, he often hopped up and down, and he frequently slid from corner to corner on the small conductor's podium.

Both symphony players and audience feared that one day he would surely fall off the podium and kill himself. Toscanini shared that fear, especially after the famous English composer and impresario Sir Thomas Beecham fell off the podium while subbing for him at a New York Philharmonic rehearsal. Conductor's shoes in those days had smooth leather soles. In combination with a typical polished wooden podium, falling was an ever-present danger.

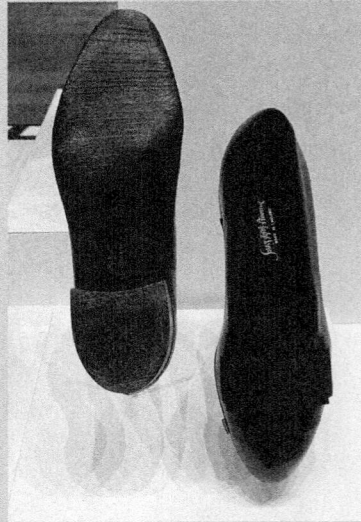

Toscanini commissioned Saks Fifth Avenue to alter his shoes in a manner that would reduce his risk of a fatal fall. Saks passed the job on to a well-known British shoemaker who took a pair of smooth-soled shoes and scored the soles and heels to make them slip resistant (fig. 13). His bespoke shoes along with a full explanation are on display at (of all places) the New York Public Library.

Figure 13. Toscanini's shoes. The scoring consists mostly of parallel shallow grooves that roughen the sole and heel, thus increasing the kinetic coefficient of friction. Mission accomplished—Toscanini never fell off the podium.

TOSCANINI'S SHOES CONT'D.

Today, conductor podiums are covered with a non-slip surface. I doubt that was an option when Toscanini considered what to do about his risk of falling.

Performers are always at risk from falling off the stage. Recently, Ian McKellen, the most famous English actor of our day, fell off a stage. He claims that matters could have been worse had he not been wearing a padded suit to make him look like Falstaff. Despite his seemingly minor injuries, persistent pain has essentially prevented this cultural icon from returning to the stage.

multiple microchannels and canals to carry water away, much like special running shoes. This feature increases the dry surface area of their feet, which adds to the effective COF. Penguins also waddle slowly from side-to-side, reflecting their need to keep their center of gravity low by planting their entire foot down. Taking small penguin steps is a good way to avoid falling on ice.

So far, I have confined my discussion to walking on ice. But a typical day in or out of the house offers many unsuspecting places where you might encounter slippery surfaces. These need to be addressed as diligently as a stroll on ice.

In many eastern countries, shoes must be removed in the home and at a house of worship. In Japan, outdoor shoes are removed at the genkan, an entryway area to a house, apartment, or building, and where one usually dons indoor slippers. Removing shoes at home and a house of worship is common in many other eastern countries as well.

Wearing socks without shoes in a house with waxed wooden floors greatly increases your risk of a fall.

We previously discussed the slipperiness of showers and tubs, as well as outside flooring such as granite and marble. Any smooth surface, such as linoleum or vinyl flooring in a kitchen, can become slippery if water gets on it. It is good practice to check your and your parents' home for areas where one could slip on a polished surface, and find ways to prevent an accident.

The **fifth** way to mitigate these problems at home or in public settings is to treat the walking surface, thereby increasing the COF. In commercial settings, the Occupational Safety and Health Administration (OSHA) recommends a minimum COF of 0.5 on all surfaces. The Americans with Disabilities Act (ADA) goes further, recommending a COF of 0.6 on flat surfaces and 0.8 on ramps. Nonethless, these remain guidelines only.

Tribology is the science of measuring the static and kinetic COFs in various settings, not just at home; a tribometer is an extremely sensitive device used to measure the COF of two materials. You may be surprised to learn that tribologists are in great demand in industry, where friction is sometimes your friend but more often your enemy, because friction generates massive amounts of useless heat. The word tribology derives from the Greek word τριβή, meaning friction. It sounds like it's related to the English word trip. It isn't, but it seems like it should be.

Appendix B offers a more mathy look at penguin steps if you're interested in these sorts of things.

CHAPTER 9

Information from a Variety of Sources

The web is full of facts and advice related to falls. We already observed in the introduction how demographics—the study of a population's age, sex, and race, for example—no matter how important to the study of falls, sheds little useful light on fall prevention.

Several sites give detailed instructions on how to protect yourself when you fall. Two web pages emphasize taking care to fall in a gentle manner, always protecting vulnerable body parts of your body from injury. [34,35] That does not describe the way I, and I suspect most individuals, fall. I go from standing to fully crumpled in what seems like a millisecond, leaving little time to strategize the finer points of getting into the most favorable position, one of which, unlikely outside a banana peel trip, is to land on your *prat* (another word for bum)—hence the word *pratfall*. Better to prevent a fall in the first place than minimize its effects.

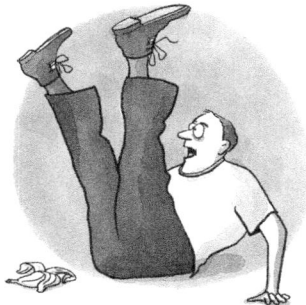

CHAPTER 10

Medications and Falls

Few people I know have significantly reduced the number of meds they take daily. I'm constantly trying to rearrange the meds in my medicine cabinet to accommodate their ever increasing number, although some enlightened physicians now advocate "deprescribing" as many as possible.[36]

Many categories of medications have properties that could potentially lead to a fall.[37] Medications come with inserts that list potential side effects. Like me, you probably discard them promptly because they are either printed in too small a font, look boring, or physically get in the way of accessing them.

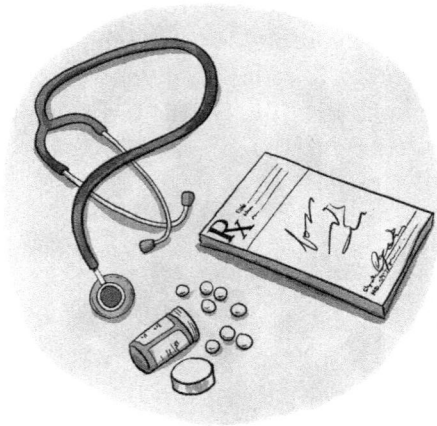

If you read the side-effects section of all the prescription and over-the-counter medications you take, you will probably find one or more that list **fatigue, drowsiness, and lightheadedness** as a side effect, especially if you're taking sleeping pills, sedatives, or anti-hypertensives. That's why I take all my meds, including my sleeping pills and antihypertensives just before I go to bed.* If perchance I die before I wake, then my wife will surely understand why. Since she always goes to sleep before me, my last words on earth will be "No problem", after her invariable reminder to turn out the lights in the TV room before going upstairs to bed.

The three categories in bold above are highly correlated with medication-associated falls and their adverse effects are mostly additive. In a government issued toolkit designed to measure medication related fall risk, three points are given to each analgesic, anti-psychotic, anticonvulsant, and benzodiazepine you take; two points each are given to antihypertensives, cardiac drugs, antiarrhythmics, and antidepressants; one point is given to a diuretic.[38] If the sum is greater than six, then you are at high risk for a fall. The next time you visit your physician, ask if you are taking too many of these types of pills.

In the elderly, two commonly prescribed medication classes are notably associated with falls, namely benzodiazepines (street name—*benzos, downers*) and antihypertensives.

All benzodiazepine drugs produce some degree of sedation. In general, short-acting benzodiazepines, such as temazepam (Restoril), are used as sleeping pills, and long-acting benzodiazepines are used to treat anxiety. Short-acting benzodiazepines tend to be addictive. Many senior citizens struggle with insomnia and thus depend on sleeping pills, which render them increasingly likely to fall.

It is easy to confuse the class of medication, *benzodiazepines*, with the similar sounding brand name medication, Benadryl. And

---

*Recently, my Harvard Medical School health bulletin published the results of a randomized controlled study of whether the time of day you take your pills makes a difference in your incidence of stroke or heart attack after five years. Bottom line—it doesn't.

not to mention a "Benny", which is slang for Benzedrine, a common amphetamine widely used around 1960. That's just the opposite of a sleeping pill.

The primary use of the antihistamine Benadryl is to treat allergies, but it is also commonly used alone or in combination with over-the-counter pain medications such as in Tylenol PM, Advil PM, and Aleve PM, with the PM representing the use of Benadryl as an aid for insomnia. The risk profile of Benadryl is way better than that of Restoril (a benzodiazepine), but then again, it is far less effective than a sleeping pill.

I don't want to leave you with the impression that medications have only the potential to cause harm. Bone is a living tissue that constantly breaks down and is replaced. Osteoporosis is a condition in which the bones become brittle and fail to keep up with the replacement process.

There are many risk factors associated with osteoporosis, such as age (more common in the frail elderly), female sex, and hormone imbalance.

Osteoporosis-related fractures are common in the elderly and often involve the hip. Obviously, it is best to diagnose and treat the disease before a fall, since the baneful outcome of a fall in a person with osteoporosis is significantly greater than otherwise. A simple bone density test establishes the diagnosis, and many medications are available to treat the condition. You should request that your physician order that test every five years or so.

The truth of this policy is best illustrated with an example. Bernie Salick, MD, is a successful eighty-seven-year-old physician-entrepreneur who started his medical career as a nephrologist (kidney specialist) in 1970, about five years before I finished my post-graduate studies in vascular surgery. Shortly after Bernie started practicing, Medicare began to cover the prohibitive cost of dialysis care in patients with kidney failure, which typically results from advanced diabetes and hypertension. Kidney dialysis requires treatment three times a week, and at first, African American patients struggled to travel to dialysis centers, which were often located in affluent neighborhoods far from where they lived. Few physicians were willing to travel to south-central LA to provide care.

Bernie decided to take this new treatment to the patients. He built many dialysis centers in south-central Los Angeles and quickly became a financial success. Years later, Bernie took his entrepreneurial skills to Cedars-Sinai Medical Center and he established the Sam Ochsin Cancer Center. Along the way Bernie also became a celebrated philanthropist.

Bernie and I share a primary care physician, Hector Rodriguez, who is chief of nephrology at Cedars. I received my post-medical school surgical training there, and it's where Bernie and I spent our entire careers. Cedars is now a world-renowned teaching and research hospital.

Hector discovered that Bernie had profound osteoporosis about a year ago and so he treated him aggressively. I would like to believe that Hector had read the early version of *The Fall Guy* I gave him, and that he was thus inspired to test and then treat Bernie for osteoporosis. Recently, while visiting Cedars on an unrelated matter, Bernie fell down a flight of stairs and fractured his skull. He remained in a coma for one week and has since been recovering slowly but steadily. Hector believes Bernie would have died had he not been treated for osteoporosis the previous year.

I never encountered a problem with the many pain pills I prescribed in my practice, but I often saw patients in whom initiating or increasing the dosage of an antihypertensive medication caused an unacceptably low blood pressure, resulting in lightheadedness and occasionally a fall.

High blood pressure is an important risk factor for stroke and hardening of the arteries, and low blood pressure poses the risk of falling. Physicians who prescribe antihypertensives are constantly challenged to establish and maintain the correct dosage—neither too much nor too little. Furthermore complicating the medical provider's task, the prescription guidelines seem to change frequently.

For instance, a recent study[39] concluded that most individuals over eighty could get by with a blood pressure of 160 systolic (the upper number of the two) or less, which is higher than the 140 recommended for younger individuals.

These sad truths affected my own mother. She was in excellent health when I received a call from her internist, a professor of medicine at Northwestern University. He told me that her blood pressure had been very low and she was experiencing dizziness. She had undergone extensive testing and he could not explain why her pressure was so low. He felt he should give her medicine that would raise her blood pressure. Of course, I agreed, but the mystery of it all made me very uncomfortable.

One year later he called again to tell me that my mother was found unconscious and was rushed to the ER. A CT scan showed a bleed into her brain. Such bleeds often occur when the blood pressure is very high, but he could not tell me if the high blood pressure was from the new medicine or the fact that blood pressure can arise just from bleeding into the brain.

I immediately flew to Chicago and the internist suggested I review the CT scan before seeing my mother. One look at the scan told me she would never again be the mother I adored. The bleed had practically filled half her skull and I couldn't believe she was still alive.

I went to her bedside where she was conscious and talking, but not making much sense. I predicted either a poor recovery or none at all. Regrettably, she also had significant memory loss, declined slowly over several years, and eventually passed away.

Everyone should own a home blood pressure monitor. You should check your pressure frequently during the first couple of weeks after any change in the dosage of your antihypertensive or sedatives. Report pressures at or below ninety systolic. Next time you have an office appointment with your doctor, an ever-infrequent event these days, bring your home blood pressure monitor with you to check the accuracy of your device. Home monitors are seldom calibrated after they are bought.

MEDICATIONS AND FALLS

One of the most dangerous medications still in use today is Warfarin, a blood thinner whose name applies to both the branded and generic versions. Because I was a vascular surgeon, I often initiated and monitored the proper dose of that medication. Today, Warfarin is used much less often than, say, ten years ago because safer new medications are now available to prevent blood clots in a number of clinical settings.

The only common use for Warfarin today is to prevent clots from forming on the valves of patients who have an implanted artificial heart valve. The major risk of this drug is internal bleeding—dangerous enough when the bleeding is in your stomach, but often fatal when it occurs in your brain.

I include this warning about Warfarin here because I had a wonderful secretary whose mother had a mitral valve replacement. A pharmacist initiated and monitored her Warfarin dose. When she went back to the pharmacist after receiving the medication for a few days, the prothrombin test indicated that she wasn't adequately anticoagulated. The pharmacist prescribed a higher dose and asked that she return in a week.

Before the week was up, she reported a severe headache, and the prothrombin test indicated she was way over-anticoagulated. A CT scan showed a large intracerebral bleed, and she passed away shortly thereafter.

My secretary lost her mother, and I lost my secretary to depression. In some patients, the correct dosage can be exceedingly difficult to establish, as in this case.

CHAPTER 11

Time Off for Fun

Recreational injuries result in busy emergency rooms. Whether you walk, run, play tennis (my older son once tripped while jumping over the net), rollerblade, play football, ride a motorcycle, or free-climb mountains (without ropes and harnesses), you expose yourself to serious injuries of all sorts. You never know what you're going to injure when you fall.

Let's go rollerblading. The most common injuries in that sport involve the wrists, knees, and ankles. You can prevent the first two with suitable guards, but not the third. My wife is an excellent rollerblader who takes care to wear maximum gear—wrist and knee guards, and a helmet. Every time she is on the Venice bike path, she looks like a speedy armadillo. Fortunately, she has never injured herself.

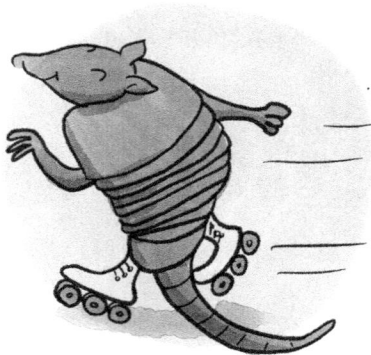

Not so with me. I fell while standing perfectly still (mentioned in the introduction) and cracked a front tooth hours before I was on tap to be the master of ceremonies at our medical fraternity's annual meeting. I looked like *Mad* magazine's Alfred E. Neuman.[40] My dentist kindly repaired the tooth in time, even though it was a Saturday.

I always marvel at the graceful movement of expert rollerbladers and ice skaters. I am also in awe at the aficionados of rollerblade hockey, who I see playing furiously without any safety equipment whatsoever. The National Hockey League justifiably goes 180 degrees on that idea. I'm sure there are some professional players who would happily play without some or almost all of their protective kit, but the team owners wisely nix that option.

At the other end of the sport spectrum, Susie and I have a friend who skydives. Half the world thinks that is the craziest sport of them all. Count us in that half. Our friend broke a leg after a routine jump and she hobbled around for two months. She promptly resumed skydiving when she healed. Like I said, some people are crazy.[41]

Falling injuries can and often do result in truly serious injuries, including death. I recall one young woman who came to the emergency room with a mangled leg following a motorcycle accident. The leg was eventually amputated after I spent eight hours trying to save it. I blamed myself and cried for days.

I am not here to tell you to stop dangerous sports, only to recommend you wear maximum gear—and always look twenty feet ahead of you.

CHAPTER 12

Watch Your Back

In this chapter I embark on a subject seldom discussed in the context of falls, namely the underappreciated role a healthy, pain-free back has in preventing them. As before, I start with my own back history to give context. And yes, I've had more than my share of afflictions in my advancing years.

About forty years ago, I joined a local gym, and being the typical doctor who knows everything about everything, I began an unsupervised exercise program that included lifting heavy weights. One day I suddenly developed excruciating back pain radiating down my left leg and into my foot. I instantly knew I had ruptured a disc and suspected an epidural would help.

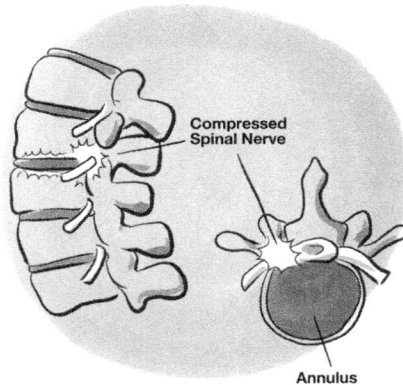

Compressed Spinal Nerve

Annulus

Let me back up briefly to explain spinal anatomy. The spine itself consists of stacked bones, collectively called vertebrae.

Between each vertebra (singular) lies a disc-shaped object called, appropriately, a disc. Think of a flattened marshmallow. Each disc consists of a tough outer membrane called an *annulus* (the Latin word meaning ring). The annulus contains a thick viscous fluid that acts like a cushion between the vertebrae. The annulus, with its contained viscous fluid allows your spine to bend.

Running down the dead center of the stacked vertebrae is a channel. This channel, or spinal canal, contains all the nerves connecting the brain with the rest of your body's anatomy, except the nerves that feed your face and other organs high up in your body.

The spinal canal is crowded. If you rupture a disc and the viscous fluid is forced out of the annulus into the canal, there's a good chance it will pinch a nerve whose function is, say, to provide sensation to a toe. Hence the agonizing pain I felt that day.

I called an anesthesiologist friend to give me an epidural, which is an injection of medication directly into the spinal canal. If it works, it reduces inflammation and the pressure on the nerve causing pain. My friend said he could do that at my home, which surprised me. He showed up and pulled out what shockingly looked like a foot long needle. He then proceeded to give me a pain-free injection that instantly relieved my agony.

The happiness of that moment lasted about a week. I called him, demanding another shot, which worked as before. After that, the pain did not rebound as much, so I rode out the ruptured disc and returned to work after about three weeks.

Fast forward twenty years, when I spontaneously ruptured a different disc. This time I needed outpatient surgery to suck out the viscous fluid.

I thought I was done with back problems. Years passed. I gradually acquired increasing pain in my back and hips and I concluded I had progressive arthritis that was getting worse hand-in-hand with my advancing age. I walked hunched over and had pain both walking and just getting out of a chair. I tolerated this state of affairs until the back and hip pain became appreciably worse.

An MRI revealed diffuse spinal stenosis, which meant my spinal canal had narrowed over a distance of three or so vertebrae due to arthritis. Since I now had access to Google and continued to insist I knew everything about everything, I concluded I would need a humongous operation to correct the spinal stenosis and relieve the pressure on my nerves. I turned to more physical therapy and epidurals, but they were a waste of time. I suspected neither would ever permanently relieve my discomfort, and I was right.

I continued to stall until the pain became intolerable and I was forced to see a spine surgeon. I crawled into Hyun Bae's office and was astonished to learn that all I needed was an outpatient operation with a high likelihood of success in helping, if not totally relieving, my back pain.

I was blown away with the result. I am now totally free of back and hip pain. Evidently even the hip pain was secondary to the spinal stenosis. I walk my four miles briskly without a scintilla of pain, and I stand erect.

I hope you can see where I am going with this. The technology of back surgery had changed dramatically in the previous ten years. Operations that previously would have kept me in bed with significant pain for weeks had now turned into a relatively pain-free microscopic outpatient procedure with rapid recovery.

It is clear, at least to me, that the surgery significantly reduced my chance of falling, since walking with pain and being continuously hunched over are definitely risk factors for falling. I confirmed the likely truth of this conjecture with Colin Stokol, MD, an accomplished neurologist and dear friend.

Even if you previously had back surgery with poor or mediocre results and you're still having back pain, it is worth checking with a neurologist or spine surgeon to see if you are a candidate for these new minimally invasive procedures.

CHAPTER 13

The Eyes Have It

The word cataract derives from the Greek prefix καταmeaning down, and was eventually used to construct the word cataract, in the sense of a waterfall. An untreated eye cataract resembles a frothy waterfall (Figure 14). If left untreated, patients go blind because the condition affects both eyes, often simultaneously. The British noticed that RAF fighter pilots who had Plexiglas embedded into their eye from shattered windshields did not get a reaction to the plastic, but US pilots who had real glass embedded in their eyes did not do so well. Thus began the era of plastic replacement of cataracts, which continues to this day. The latest advance is to implant light adjustable lenses, which brings patients closer to not needing glasses for either distance or reading.

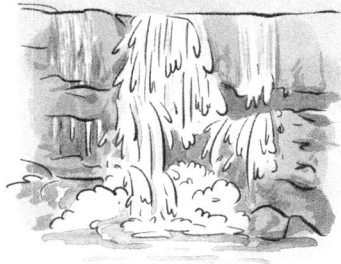

Age-related cataracts often start to develop between ages fifty to seventy. If you fall after age fifty, you should have your eyes checked, among other things. I'm guessing I was about sixty when Susie suggested I visit Nicole Fram, MD for a routine exam. She observed early cataracts and said I should return in five years. When I did, it was her opinion I should have the cataracts repaired. I was surprised because I didn't think I had a vision problem at all, and I was certain my vision hadn't changed from Dr. Fram's first examination. After I had the first cataract surgery, I realized how very wrong I was.

The repair consists of a small incision in the cornea. The cataract, which is semi-solid, is lasered, vacuumed out, and replaced with a plastic lens. Failure to repair the cataract is associated with a significant risk of falling due to blurred vision and lack of depth. I said yes to the surgery, since I knew it was a safe, outpatient procedure.

And then came the kicker. Nicole said, gently, "You know, you have epithelial membrane dystrophy in both corneas and I need to do a simple procedure on each one before you can get your cataracts fixed." Did I hear simple? I'm always on board with simple. She said, "I'll have to do it another day." I have a trusted retired ophthalmologist friend, and he said that, yes, you need to fix this condition before you can have your cataracts fixed.

So I arrived on the allotted day and Nicole numbed one eye. She returned a few minutes later with a Q-tip. Oh, this *is* simple, I thought to myself. She proceeded to roll the Q-tip over the cornea, and in a couple of minutes she was finished. I asked why she did only one eye. She chuckled and responded with "You'll see (no pun intended)". She kept me in the room for about five minutes and then said I could schedule the other eye in a couple of weeks.

All was well until I reached the elevator, at which moment I suddenly experienced intense searing pain in the treated eye. The anesthetic was short-acting and it had now worn off. If Susie hadn't been holding me by the hand, I would have crashed to the floor. This agonizing pain persisted for a few days and gradually dissipated. I was not looking forward to the second "simple" Q-tip procedure. I gritted my teeth and this time I wasn't surprised when the excruciating pain again hit after ten minutes. Epithelial membrane dystrophy is rare, as is the need to scrape the cornea before cataract surgery.

When I returned for the follow up appointment, it was time to plan for the cataract extraction, which would be done in a surgicenter.

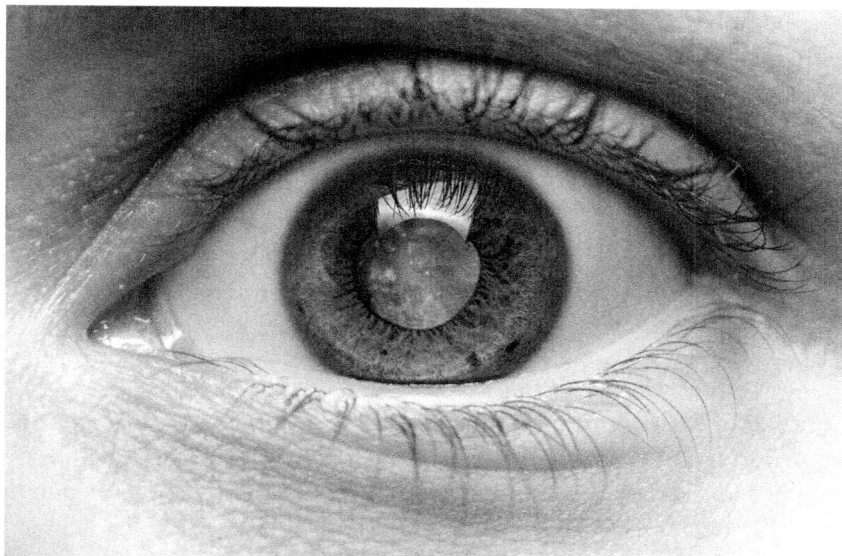

Figure 14. *This is what an untreated cataract looks like. The lens is opaque and the individual is blind in this eye. A similar untreated cataract likely is present in the other eye.*

Nicole presented me with three choices. I could have both lenses designated for reading—which meant I would need glasses for distance; or I could opt to have both lenses set for distance—which meant I would need glasses for reading; or I could have one lens for closeup and one for distance. The decision, I was told, would be permanent, because taking a lens out and replacing it with the opposite configuration has more complications than if you leave it the original way. I chose to have both lenses designed for distance, because at the time I needed to have binocular vision to use loupes (the kind you often see on TV when movies or ads portray surgeons in the operating room.)*

At the time, I didn't know I would be retiring in three years, and that after a year or so after retiring, I would come to regret my original decision (my good friend George Goldberg chose the blended

---

*It's actually a cliché because most surgeons (general, urological, orthopedic, and gynecological) don't routinely use loupes to operate.

approach and no longer needs glasses.) I still need reading glasses, and, if you know me, you would know that I forget where I put them at least three times a day.

Whichever lens configuration you prefer, it is helpful before you have cataract surgery to duplicate your future lens status with contact lenses. The doctor will need to determine the dominant and non-dominant eyes. It is imperative that if you choose "blended" vision, with one for distance and the other for near, that the dominant eye should be the distance eye every time and the doctor operate on that eye first.

After your first cataract surgery, you will notice a dramatic change of vision in the operated eye. The new lens will eliminate the yellow tint you didn't know you had, and it will provide you with significantly increased visual acuity and clarity. I simply couldn't believe I had been walking around so visually impaired. I could now compare vision in both eyes and see the difference for myself. I find it interesting that statistics convincingly show that correcting one cataract reduces the frequency of falls, but that replacing the second cataract adds nothing further to fall prevention.[42]

Nonetheless, you will want to have an operation on the other eye, if only because the yellow tint remaining in the opposite eye will be annoying (it was for me).

Macular degeneration and glaucoma are also fall risks, but only wet macular degeneration and glaucoma are easily treated.

CHAPTER 14

Playing Footsie

Foot and ankle problems are common in older folks and are associated with impaired balance and functional disability while walking. Few prospective studies, however, have been done to determine whether foot and ankle problems are indeed risk factors for falls.[43]

Fallers exhibit decreased ankle flexibility and more severe bunion deformity. Neuropathy is commonly seen in diabetics, and often occurs naturally as we age. Decreased ability to bend your toes is often genetic. Fallers are more likely to have disabling foot pain, especially in the ball and heel of the foot. Deltoid ligament* and Achilles tendon injuries lead to ankle instability. Plantar fasciitis is also a risk factor.

Foot and ankle problems do increase the risk of falls. Interventions addressing these factors may hold promise as a strategy to prevent falls.

There two good reasons to have your physician order a referral to a podiatrist and/or a physical therapist who specializes in foot and ankle problems (often found at a hospital's rehabilitation center)—if you experience a single major fall or have an intrinsic factor that affects your gait. Intrinsic factors (see the Introduction above) include Parkinson's disease, cerebral palsy, neuropathy

---

*The deltoid ligament is a strong ligament in the inner ankle area.

(inability to feel your feet) or, rarely, a missing all-important big toe, say, due to diabetes. You can do a simple test at home, called the 10 meter (25 foot) walk test to help assess your walking status.[44]

Solutions exist for reducing falls in these at-risk individual, such as wearing custom shoes, especially in those over age fifty. Custom made insoles may help as well.

CHAPTER 15

*Of Questionable Benefit
or Relevance*

Anyone who has visited a hospital either as patient or visitor cannot fail to notice the measures in place to prevent a patient from accidentally falling out of bed or while walking. Everywhere you look you see bed rails, gurneys, and walkers. Each accidental fall is reviewed at every level from the floor nurses up to top administration. And justifiably so. Although there is elevated risk of falling in a hospital, the actual incidence is quite low—between three and five per one thousand bed-days.[45]

The CDC (Centers for Disease Control and Prevention) publishes an excellent general overview—written in the form of a care plan for health care providers—of how to prevent falls in older individuals.[46]

Another excellent resource relating to falls and injury in general is the Caregiver University page of Rehabmart's website.[47] Here you will find many informative blogs as well as information comparing a wide variety of devices related to falls and other sundry conditions. As you browse, keep in mind this is a commercial website. I was particularly intrigued with products designed to raise individuals to a sitting position once they have fallen and are unable to get up without assistance. Many of these can be used at home, where they serve as a quick and inexpensive alternative to calling paramedics.

Your parents will thank you profusely if you introduce them to Skechers hands-free slip-in shoes.[48] These shoes are remarkably easy to don and provide significant comfort and support as well. They are wardrobe necessities for many older individuals, especially those with severe arthritis and back problems. I love mine.

In the special category of *Advice to Physicians Regarding Office Patients Who Fall Off Exam Tables*—surely an exceedingly small number—I once received a flash memo from my malpractice insurance carrier notifying all physicians never to leave a patient sitting on the edge of an exam table, tell her to stay put, and then walk out of the room. The cost of their insurance is less than other malpractice insurance carriers because they proactively reach out to inform doctors about measures and practices to take to avoid so-called medical mishaps—a euphemism for malpractice suits. Prospective candidates for their insurance need an up or down vote by all current members before they are approved. I was grateful that writing complete and legible medical notes wasn't a requirement for coverage.

CHAPTER 16

The History of Falls

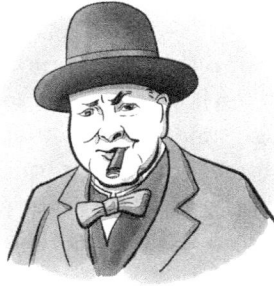

Between falls, I enjoy reading history. I am including this chapter, which I consider to be an *amuse-bouche* in the tale of fall prevention. Even if you dislike history, I encourage you to stick a toe into it. If not, move on to Chapter 17—but no refunds.

I'm dividing this chapter into two parts:

1. Famous falls *not* involving people, and
2. Falls of famous people.

I'll start with the irresistible nursery rhyme about Humpty Dumpty, who had a great fall* (fig. 15). The author of the actual ditty is unknown.

---

*Humpty Dumpty sat on a wall,
  Humpty Dumpty had a great fall,
  All the king's horses and all the king's men,
  Couldn't put Humpty back together again.

Humpty Dumpty started life as the name British Royalists (forces aligned with King Charles I) gave to a specific exceptionally large cannon during the English Civil War (1642-49).[†]

As the story goes, Parliament, which was battling the king's forces, greatly damaged the wall on which Humpty Dumpty (the cannon) had been placed. Not surprisingly, Humpty Dumpty fell, bursting into smithereens. Lewis Carroll later embellished the story and transformed the cannon into an egg in chapter VI of *Through the Looking Glass*,[49] the successor novel to *Alice's Adventures in Wonderland*.

Although the word oval literally means egg-shaped, the current use of that word applies only to a two-dimensional shape, not to Humpty Dumpty the egg.

There was no railing around the wall Humpty Dumpty was sitting on and he rolled off after Alice left him at the end of the chapter. A loud crash resounded through the forest. All the king's horses and all the king's men suddenly appeared at the request of the king, presumably to put Humpty Dumpty back together again. Ironically, many of the king's men themselves fell down, resulting in little heaps of them.

Well, we all know that the horses never had a chance to put Humpty Dumpty back together again because they have hooves, not prehensile (grasping) fingers, as we humans do.

Once Humpty Dumpty fell and his innards "scrambled," there was no chance *anyone* could ever put him back together again. If you instinctively understand that, you instinctively understand the second law of thermodynamics. Scientists use the second law to predict the ultimate fate of our universe, which is that everything in our universe will eventually become homogeneous. The process of becoming homogeneous can be calculated, and the result is a number (entropy) which ranges between zero and one, with one representing maximum disorder. Entropy always gets bigger in any closed system, which our universe presumably is.[‡]

[†] Almost all nursery rhymes have historical roots.

[‡] A closed system in one in which you neither add nor subtract energy.

See what you can learn from a nursery rhyme?

Then there's hapless Jack, who fell down a hill breaking his crown, and Jill, who fell down after him.

Here's a short list of famous individuals who fell to their death, or just fell a lot. Although that list includes the death of William the Conqueror, he hardly counts for the purposes of this book, since falling off a horse is hardly preventable, unless you consider his extreme corpulence as a contributing factor.

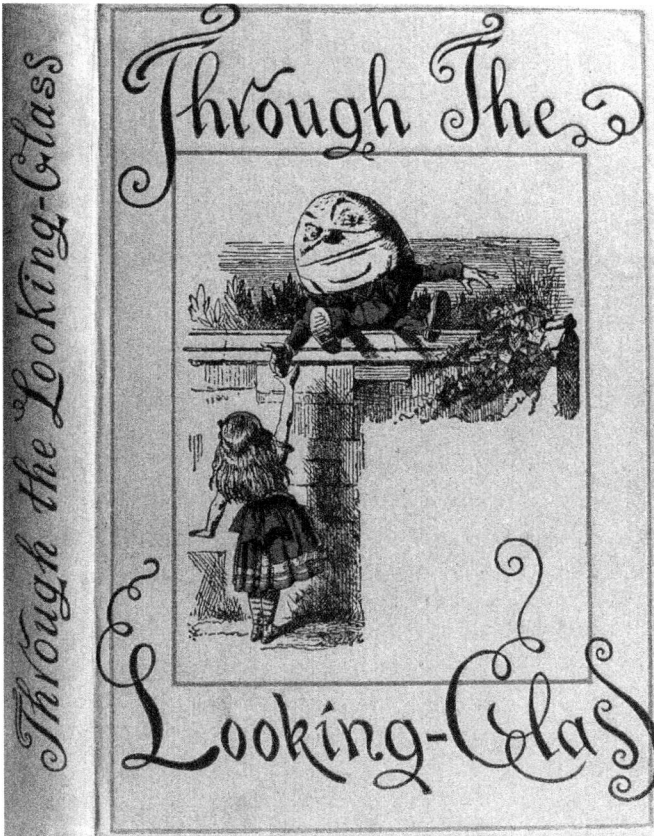

Figure 15. *Alice shakes hands with Humpty Dumpty in Chapter VI of "Through the Looking Glass" by Lewis Carroll. The caricaturist John Tenniel created this iconic image.*

One well-known individual who died of a head injury after a fall is Joseph Lieberman (1942–2024), a beloved State of Connecticut politician. Throughout his career he stubbornly chose centrist over partisan politics. He was, uniquely, elected the Connecticut state senator as both Democrat and independent and he even endorsed the Republican candidate, John McCain, in the 2008 presidential election.[50]

Finally, I would like to introduce you to the patron saint of falls and accidents, none other than Sir Winston Churchill (1874–1965), quite likely the greatest political leader of the twentieth century.

His physical falls[51] began when he fell off his tricycle at age five and fell off his bicycle later at Harrow. In 1893, while playing a game of chase, he jumped off a footbridge, trusting that the branches in the trees below would cushion his fall. They didn't. After falling thirty feet, he experienced the effects of a concussion for three days, ruptured a kidney,[§] and broke a bone in his back, which was not detected for years.

Shortly after joining the 4th Queen's Own Hussars, a cushy military assignment, he ruptured his sartorius muscle (a key muscle in the thigh), and was later thrown off his horse while steeple chasing. He accepted a challenging position in India. At the end of his voyage to Bombay, today's Mumbai, he reached for an iron ring just as his landing boat shifted position. This resulted in a chronically painful dislocated right shoulder, which greatly affected his ability to play polo and tennis. A few months later he fell from a pony and injured his left shoulder. And then a bullet misfired leaving shards in his hand. He was still a young man.

In the middle of a three-year hiatus between personal injuries, it might seem churlish to relate details surrounding the death of Churchill's mother, Lady Randolph (Jeanette) Churchill. She had recently

---

[§] A medical school classmate fell and also ruptured a kidney. Like Churchill, he was treated nonoperatively because in contrast to the spleen, the kidney is surrounded by a very strong capsule which confines the bleeding to a small volume. Football players wear "kidney pads" to prevent injury in that area.

purchased dainty ultra-tall Italian high-heeled shoes and fell down a short flight stairs, fracturing her ankle. The lower leg became massively swollen and then gangrenous. The decision was made to amputate at the mid-thigh level. Several days later, the ligature securing the thigh artery loosened. The thigh wound hemorrhaged, resulting in her rapid demise.¶

There was no respite from his own injuries, however. Years after these events, Churchill fell victim to the common Englishman's error of looking in the wrong direction while crossing the street.** Churchill always considered himself bi-national because he had an American mother and an English father. Although he had previously visited America many times, he got halfway across Fifth Avenue, looked left when he should have looked right, and got slammed. He experienced yet another concussion and broken toes. He recovered quickly, however, and gave the driver of the car a signed copy of his book, *The Eastern Front*.

Three years before he died at age 90, Churchill fell in Monaco and fractured his left hip and femur. He was hospitalized for fifty-five days. Mercifully, this was his last major injury.

¶ To a vascular surgeon like me, this sequence of events, at first, seems fantastical knowing the then-current excellent state of surgical practice in post WWI England. Surgeons could easily handle a thigh amputation without such a catastrophic complication. Her initial injury was most likely a Jones fracture—which results from a sudden inward twist of the foot—when she crashed coming down the stairs. Jones fractures are notoriously associated with gangrene of the fifth toe. She should not have been wearing high heel shoes because she was now overweight and probably not holding on to a banister. If her doctor had told her to elevate her leg at all times, the swelling in her foot would have receded, and the worst that would happen is that only her gangrenous toe would need to be amputated. Limb amputation became a routine operation ever since Ambroise Paré (1510-1590), who is often called the Father of Modern Surgery, published how to perform complication-free amputations.

** Of course, this mistake is not confined to the English, as the author of this book can readily attest.

CHAPTER 17

The Takeaway

Here is what I'd like you to take away from this book. I divide that picture into three categories. The first includes measures to prevent bad falls, like following the twenty-foot rule, putting strips of tape on steps, lighting the path from your front door to the sidewalk, and buying Skechers hands-free slip-in shoes.

The second includes efforts to stay healthy, like diet and exercise. They do not play an overarching role in preventing falls, but even the moderate exerciser and weight loser is way ahead of anyone who makes no effort to do either.

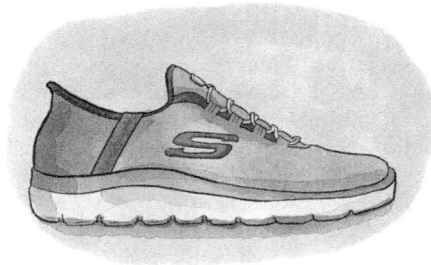

The third involves the theme of mental awareness. I have learned the hard way that to prevent falls, you need to be constantly alert. And you need to Think Awareness, whether you are old, active in sports, or doing anything, really. Anticipation is crucially important.

Consider driving. It's not enough to know the laws and how to drive. You must constantly watch out for the other driver and know how to react prophylactically to ward off an accident (e.g., the idiot who cuts you off, and the driver who makes a mistake or brakes suddenly in front of you).

If you are of a certain age, you should not be so proud to think you don't need to sit to put on your shoes and socks. Talk prevention with your partner, and encourage each other to do the right thing.

Someone who doesn't wear a helmet while riding a motorcycle or who walks while her eyes are locked onto her cellphone screen (see front cover) isn't seriously tuned into the possibility of injury. The assumption that "it will never happen to me" is an approach shared with an ostrich. It boils down to common sense and being vigilant at all times.

CHAPTER 18

Platform shoes

If you bought this book to get advice on this topic, you are either extremely mentally dense or you have rubber bones. Enough said. Oh—and don't get me started on falls secondary to good bourbon.

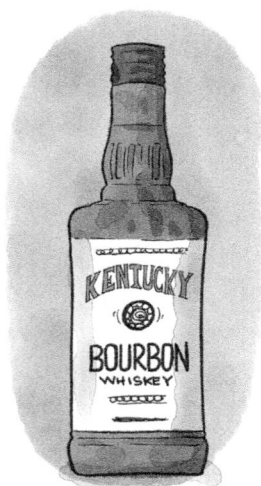

APPENDIX A

Exercises to Prevent Falls

These exercises are organized into a group of five that you do standing, and two groups that you do flat on your back with a small pillow beneath your head. I suggest doing them consistently three to four times per week. I believe that the law of diminishing returns sets in quickly when it comes to exercise, so doing them more often does not add substantial benefit. If you can't do the recommended number of repetitions, do as many as you can and work your way up. If you are truly pressed for time, I recommend doing the squats, lunges, and the last group of hip exercises.

STANDING

Squats. Put two hands on the edge of a cabinet, wall, or chair to maintain balance.

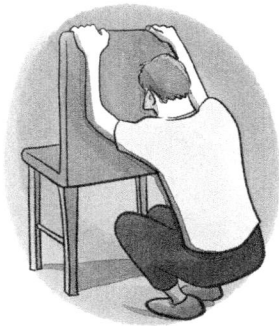

If you already have moderately good balance, place a long plastic rod behind your neck and hold it with both hands. Either way, squat down as far as your knees will allow. Repeat ten times. The main purpose of this exercise is to strengthen your quads and glutes, which kick in when you rise from the squat. The slower you get up from the squat, the more burn you will feel. The stronger your quads and glutes, the less likely you are to fall. The balance part is a bonus.

Calf Muscle Stretches. Stand erect about a foot in front of a wall, chair or cabinet. Place your hands on the wall and bring one leg back as far back you can, making sure both heels remain flat on the ground. When you lean into the wall, keep your back straight. Alternate sides for a total of ten times. This is strictly a stretch exercise for your calf muscles. Progress is measured slowly over weeks by the incremental increase in the distance you can move your leg back.

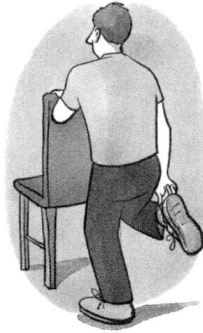

Lunges. With your arms held straight in front of you, bring one leg forward and lower your body as far down as you can. The goal of this exercise is similar to full squats, but here you are also challenging your balance more. Alternate legs by moving forward. Do twenty if you can.

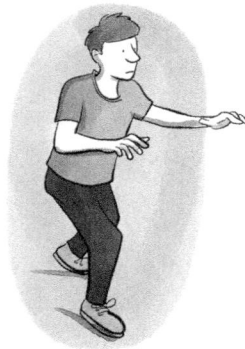

Quadriceps stretch. The quadriceps muscle is the one in the front of your thigh. Hold on to a counter top or wall for balance. Reach behind you and grab the inside of the back of the sock or shoe with two fingers on that side. Try to bring your foot up to your glutes. This exercise also benefits your knees.

Bend your leg back at the hip as much as possible. Stand straight if you can. Hold for ten seconds each side.

Stand on one foot at a time. This balance exercise is best done in a narrow corridor with carpets so that if you fall in either direction you won't hurt yourself . Try this for about ten seconds if you can, then switch to the other foot. Repeat for a second round.

LYING ON THE FLOOR

Abdominal Exercises. The following four exercises are designed to improve the stability and strength of your core (the central part of your body). (1) With your knees slightly bent, raise your buttocks off the floor, squeeze your abdominal muscles and hold for a count of ten.

Repeat twice. (2) With your knees slightly bent and your hands behind your head, do regular crunches (partial sit-ups). Try to do forty if you can. (3) Then do twenty cross crunches, ten each side. Keep your hands behind your head. Bring each elbow across to touch the raised contralateral knee. Alternate legs. (4) Finally, bend your knees, elevate your hips off the ground, and then contract your lower abdominal muscles and glutes for a count of three. Do this three times.

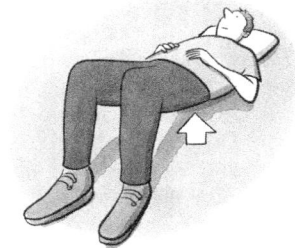

Exercises to increase hip flexibility (very important!). (1) Bend your left knee and bring it as close to your chest as possible, using both hands to increase the stretch.* (2) With your right knee slightly bent, rotate your left hip out and bring your left foot up to rest on your right knee. Use both hands to push your left knee out as much as possible.

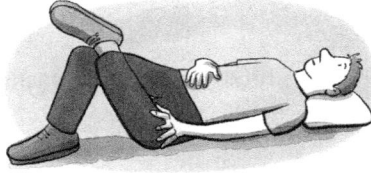

(3) Finally, raise your left leg as far as possible, taking care not to bend your knee, even if you're able to raise your leg only a few inches off the floor. Don't cheat on this one. This exercise is designed to strengthen the thigh and hip muscles and to increase the flexibility and range of motion of the hip joint.

Repeat this last set of three exercises five times on each side. This set is the most important of all, with lunges and squats running a close tie for second. How so? For the same reason Novak Djokovic is the best tennis player ever. You might think he exercises by running, lifting weights, or even playing tennis, but actually, he mostly stretches. To return the ball when it appears he could never get near it, he *stretches* into unimaginably contorted positions that astound even his opponents. Nothing gets past him.

When you encounter a situation in which a fall seems inevitable, you have a better chance of dancing around the problem with the flexibility you gain by stretching.

---

*The Japanese eat with their knees bent beneath them. This is the seiza position, or what we in the west call sitting on one's haunches, which is really a misnomer, since your haunches must rest on your heels, not the other way around. This position requires extreme knee flexion that must be acquired with practice. This first exercise tries to attain extreme knee flexion, so in theory, you could eventually eat the way the Japanese do. After several years of doing this exercise, I am still about three inches away from having my heels touch my prat (see chapter 17) when I am on my back, yet when I sit up and assume the seiza position, my haunches actually touch my heels, but my knees hurt so much that I immediately exit that position. Older Japanese men also have difficulty maintaining the Seiza position. When I first started doing this exercise, my haunches couldn't go down to touch my heels as they do now, which, to me, means I'm making slow, slow progress. At least I'm not getting worse, and that is the purpose of all stretching exercises.

APPENDIX B (OPTIONAL)

The Physics of Baby Steps

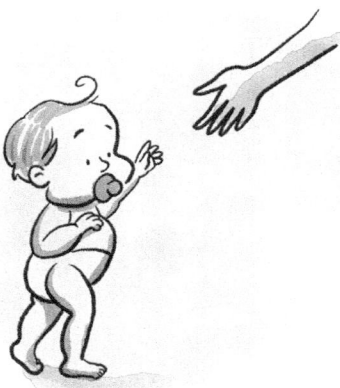

Friction is a force that always exists between two surfaces that are in contact. Microscopic observation shows that both surfaces have asperities, which are irregularities in the surface of each that create a force opposing motion. If you would like to move an object (say, a book) and it's sitting on a flat surface like a table, the force of friction acts *opposite* the direction you would like the object to move. That resistance to movement is proportional to the book's weight. If you double the weight of the book, you double the friction. For technical purposes, physicists prefer to use the concept of a normal force instead of the weight. When one object rests on top of a table or the ground, gravity is always trying to pull it toward the center of the earth. If the object is *not* moving, there must be an equal force acting in the opposite direction that keeps the object immobile, otherwise the book would fall through the table due to the earth's gravity. In physics, that force is called the normal force, or N, and is equal to the weight of the object. *

When you first start to pull (or push) the object, it may not budge. Once your pull exceeds a certain maximum, however, the object you are pulling on suddenly begins to move, and to keep the object moving, you will discover that you need to pull with a force that is *less* than the last pulling force you needed to get it moving in the first place. The force you needed *just before* the object moved is called the maximum static force (because until that moment nothing was moving) and the force you need *after* the object moves is called the kinetic, or *slipping* force, which remains constant if you are pulling the object at a constant speed. Note that the COF of a static object is usually greater than when it is in motion.

TABLE 2

	μ_s	μ_k
Ice on ice	0.10	0.03
Steel on ice	0.14	0.03
Rubber on ice	0.15	0.15
Leather on wood	0.35	0.30
Rubber on wet concrete	0.70	0.58
Rubber on wood	0.70	0.60
Rubber on dry concrete	0.90	0.68

The normal force is equivalent to but directed opposite the object's

---

*The word normal in this setting unintuitively means perpendicular to something else. Why Roman carpenters chose give the word norma to a carpenter's T-square is anyone's guess.

weight (i.e., upwards). The weight (or equivalent normal force pointed upward) of the object remains the same in both the static and moving scenarios, so it follows that the COF must be less in the kinetic state than the static state, since you are successfully pulling with less force than just before the object "gave". This finding is consistent with the values listed in Table 2 and Amonton's first law of friction, which is that the **force** required to move one object over another is the **COF x the normal force (N),** which is the same value as the weight of the object.

THE FORCE (F) REQUIRED TO MOVE ONE OBJECT OVER ANOTHER = COF X N, WHETHER AT REST OR IF THE OBJECT IS MOVING.

With this additional background to the laws of friction, it is now possible to provide a somewhat more vigorous explanation of why baby steps are essential for walking on ice.

If you take a big step on ice with your right foot, the forward component of force of your step (the thrust) may exceed the maximum static COF times your weight. If the force of your step does exceed the maximum μ_s x N calculation, you will slip and fall because the forward component of force of your step exceeded μ_k x N. This logic applies equally to the left leg if it is still on the ground. The friction in that leg is directed forward in an attempt to keep the left leg from sliding backwards. If both legs slip, your chances of staying erect vanish. Taking baby steps assures that the forward and backward forces you supply to each leg are small enough to keep the static COF from becoming a kinetic COF. Thus, the COF of either leg and underlying ice combination never exceeds the maximum static COF, which is what you want if you don't want to slip and fall.

Table 2 also explains part of the reason why anti-lock brake systems (ASB) work well in many but not all slippery conditions. An ASB systems kicks in when you jam on your brakes in an emergency.

The ASB system senses that condition, and then alternately locks and unlocks your brakes up to twenty times per second, much faster than you can do yourself. Look at the various COFs for rubber on wet and dry concrete and rubber on ice. When you drive in dry conditions, your wheels are rolling, not sliding. The applicable μ is therefore μ_s, because as the wheel turns, the only part of the wheel in contact with the concrete is not moving—it's static. If you're going slow enough and you slam on your brakes, you will stop because your velocity did not exceed the maximum COF. If you are travelling faster, your car will skid when you slam on the brakes, because you are exceeding the μ_R. This situation is much like the book on the table, except you *don't* want the car to slip (skid). In effect, When you skid, you have dropped the COF from 0.90 to 0.68. That's where ASB comes into action. It alternates rapidly between a condition where the wheel is not turning (μ_R = 0.68) and one where the wheel is turning (μ_s = 0.90). When the wheel is turning, it can take advantage of the higher COF to grip the concrete, which in turn allows the car to stop sooner, thus shortening the skid.

The argument also applies in wet conditions, in which the μ_s = 0.70 and the μ_R = 0.58. The difference between the COFs is less, but the ASB brakes will still offer a shorter skid distance than just slamming down on the brakes without the benefit of ASB.

But now look what happens when you slam on your brakes while driving on ice. Both the μ_s, and μ_R are 0.15. Whether the brakes are locked or not, your car skids and ASB brakes will not affect the length of the skid.

ENDNOTES

Introduction

1. Isaacs, Bernie. 1992. *The Challenge of Geriatric Medicine*. Oxford: Oxford University Press.

2. Jia, Haomiao et al. "Prevalence, risk factors, and burden of disease for falls and balance or walking problems among older adults in the U.S." *Preventive Medicine* vol. 126 (September, 2019): 105737. https://doi.org/10.1016/j.ypmed.2019.05.025.

3. C. Colon-Emeric, MD, MHS et.al. JAMA "Risk Assessment and Prevention of Falls in Older Community-Dwelling Adults" March 27, 2024. https://doi.org/10.100/jama.2024:1416.

Chapter 1

4. https://www.guideone.com/slips-and-falls

5. Markham Heid. "When You Stroll and Scroll, Hazards Abound", *New York Times*, January 23, 2024.

Chapter 2

6. https://safetyculture.com/topics/ladder-safety/10-ladder-safety-rules/

Chapter 3

7. https://www.bluezones.com/dan-buettner/

8. https://www.akti.org/the-useful-sword-cane/

9. https://fashionablecanes.com/collections/flask-canes

10. https://www.rehabmart.com/post/walking-canes-how-to-choose-the-best-one-for-you/

Chapter 4

11. Tsang, William W N, and Christina W Y Hui-Chan. "Effect of 4- and 8-wk intensive Tai Chi Training on balance control in the elderly." *Medicine and science in sports and exercise* vol. 36,4 (2004): 648-57. https://doi.org/10.1249/01.mss.0000121941.57669.bf

12. Granacher, Urs et al. "The performance of balance exercises during daily tooth brushing is not sufficient to improve balance and muscle strength in healthy older adults." *BMC geriatrics* vol. 21,1 257. 17 Apr. 2021. https://doi.org/doi:10.1186/s12877-021-02206-w

13. https://www.thegreatcoursesplus.com/

ENDNOTES

Chapter 5

14. Mitchell, Rebecca J et al. "Associations between obesity and overweight and fall risk, health status and quality of life in older people." *Australian and New Zealand journal of public health* vol. 38, 1 (2014): 13-8. https//doi.org/10.1111/1753-6405.12152

15. Herman Pontzer, PhD, Burn: New Research Blow the Lid off How we Really Burn Calories, Lose Weight, and Stay Healthy (New York: Penguin, 2021).

16. The basal metabolic rate (BMR), not to be confused with the body mass index (BMI).

17. Dipla, Konstantina et al. "Relative energy deficiency in sports (RED-S): elucidation of endocrine changes affecting the health of males and females." Hormones (Athens, Greece) vol. 20,1 (2021): 35-47. https://doi.org/10.1007/s42000-020-00214-w.

18. Yannakoulia, Mary, and Nikolaos Scarmeas. "Diets." *The New England journal of medicine* vol. 390,22 (2024): 2098-2106. https://doi.org/10.1056/NEJMra2211889. This manuscript discusses the composition of a number of popular diets, including Mediterranean, vegetarian, low-fat, carbohydrate-restricted (Atkins, ketogenic, and "paleo"), low-glycemic index, DASH, and fasting. Each of them has a variable effect on weight reduction and associated health benefits and each can be useful in a variety of clinical settings.

19. Shan, Zhilei et al. "Healthy Eating Patterns and Risk of Total and Cause-Specific Mortality." *JAMA internal medicine* vol. 183,2 (2023): 142-153. https://doi:10.1001/jamainternmed.2022.6117

20. Lincoff, A Michael et al. "Semaglutide and Cardiovascular Outcomes in Obesity without Diabetes." *The New England journal of medicine* vol. 389,24 (2023): 2221-2232. https://doi.org/10.1056/NEJMoa2307563

Chapter 6

21. Startzell, J K et al. "Stair negotiation in older people: a review." *Journal of the American Geriatrics Society* vol. 48,5 (2000): 567-80. https://doi.org/10.1111/j.1532-5415.2000.tb05006.x

22. J Horauf et. al. "Injury Patterns after Falling down Stairs—High Ratio of Traumatic Brain Injury under Alcohol Influence". *Journal of Clinical Medicine* 11(3); January 28, 2002:697. https://doi.org/10.3390/jcm11030697

23. https://www.dir.ca.gov/title8/1626.html

24. For my bias confirmation, see https://triskeleheritage.triskelepublishing.com/mediaeval-mythbusting-blog-2-the-man-who-invented-the-spiral-staircase-myth/. Jump to points 3 and 7 in the author's analysis of this issue.

25. https://en.wikipedia.org/wiki/Medieval_fortification

Chapter 7

26. D. H. Kim, and K Rockwood. "Frailty in Older Adults." N Engl J Jed 2024;391:538-548. https://doi.org/10.1056/NEJMra2301292. 2

27. E. Weiss et. al. "Effects of Weight Loss on Lean Mass, Strength, Bone, and Aerobic Capacity". *Med Sci in Sports Exerc.* 49(1); January, 2017:206-17. https://doi.org/10.1249/MSS.0000000000001074

ENDNOTES

Chapter 8

28. Bruijn, Sjoerd M, and Jaap H van Dieën. "Control of human gait stability through foot placement." *Journal of the Royal Society, Interface* vol. 15,143 (2018): 20170816. https://doi.org/10.1098/rsif.2017.0816

29. Andersen, Charlotte Uggerhøj et al. "Prevalence of medication-related falls in 200 consecutive elderly patients with hip fractures: a cross-sectional study." *BMC geriatrics* vol. 20,1 121. 30 Mar. 2020, https://doi.org/10.1186/s12877-020-01532-9

30. Megan Thilking. "Don't Let Your Winter Walk End Up on a Blooper Reel", *New York Times,* January 31, 2024.

31. The following animal vignettes are adapted from V. Richhariya et. al. (2023). "Unravelling the physics and mechanisms behind slips and falls on icy surfaces: A comprehensive review and nature-inspired solutions". *Materials & Design.* 234;October, 2023: 112335. https://doi.org/10.1016/j.matdes.2023

32. https://www.google.com/search?q=video+of+bouching+seals+you+tube&client=firefox-b-1-d&sca_esv=e561d0ec59a4f4d7&sca_upv=1&ei=Bs6GZpjBE-qvLuvQPuqmZ2AU&ved=0ahUKEwiY3L6p542HAxWrpY4IHbpUBlsQ4dUDC-BA&uact=5&oq=video+of+bouching+seals+you+tube&gs_lp=Egxnd3Mtd2l6LXNlcnAiIHZpZGVvIG9mIGJvdWNoaW5nIHNlYWxzIHlvdSBodWJlIMgQQIRgKSPY-fUJgJWOcRcAF4AZABAJgBVqABrASqAQE3uAEDyAEA-AEBmAIIoALLBMIC-ChAAGLADGNYEGEfCAggQABiABBiiBMICCBAAGKIEGIkFmAMA4gMFEgEEx-IECIBgGQBgiSBwE4oAe8FQ&sclient=gws-wiz-serp#fpstate=ive&vld=cid:5ac5d-9dc,vid:A4MU5BXPGcw,st:0

33. Song et al., 2018, Cell Reports 25, 2981–2991 December 11, 2018 ª 2018. https://doi.org/10.1016/j.celrep.2018.11.017

Chapter 9

34. Jen Murphy. "If You're Going to Fall Down, This Is the Right Way", *Wall Street Journal,* November 13, 2023. https://www.wsj.com/lifestyle/fitness/senior-fall-injuries-health-judo-0df5c4c0?reflink=integratedwebview/

35. Justin Barnes. "How to Fall Safely". February 23, 2023. https://www.wikihow.com/Fall-Safely/

Chapter 10

36. Leslie Kernisan. "Deprescribing: How to Be on Less Medication for Healthier Aging." https://betterhealthwhileaging.net/deprescribing-how-to-be-on-less-medication-in-aging/

37. Andersen, Charlotte Uggerhøj et al. "Prevalence of medication-related falls in 200 consecutive elderly patients with hip fractures: a cross-sectional study." *BMC geriatrics* vol. 20,1 121. 30 Mar. 2020. https://doi.org/10.1186/s12877-020-01532-9

38. J. Tsang, et. al. "Risk of Falls and Fractures in Individuals With Cataract, Age-Related Macular Degeneration, or Glaucoma." *JAMA ophthalmology* vol. 142,2 (2024): 96-106. https://doi.org/ doi:10.1001/jamaophthalmol.2023.5858

39. https://www.eshonline.org/guidelines/2023-guidelines/

ENDNOTES

Chapter 11

40. https://en.wikipedia.org/wiki/Alfred_E._Neuman

41. R. Ciccone, et .al. The mechanism of injury and the distribution of three thousand fractures and dislocations caused by parachute jumping. Journal of Bone and Joint Surgery (American edition). 1948.

Chapter 13

42. Keay L, Ho KC, Rogers K, et al. The incidence of falls after first and second eye cataract surgery: a longitudinal cohort study. *Med J Aust.* 2022;217(2):94-99. doi:10.5694/mja2.51611

Chapter 14

43. Here are two exceptions: Al Mahrouqi MM, Vicenzino B, MacDonald DA, Smith MD. Falls and falls-related injuries in individuals with chronic ankle symptoms: a cross-sectional study. *J Foot Ankle Res.* 2023;16(1):49. Published 2023 Aug 16. doi:10.1186/s13047-023-00649-5 and Awale A, Hagedorn TJ, Dufour AB, Menz HB, Casey VA, Hannan MT. Foot Function, Foot Pain, **and** Falls in Older Adults: The Framingham Foot Study. *Gerontology.* 2017;63(4):318-324. https://doi.org/10.1159/000475710

44. https://www.physio-pedia.com/10_Metre_Walk_Test. If your tape measure is only in feet, ten meters is about 25 feet. The attached video show the man using a cane to do this test because that is how he walks. Follow the directions closely. Persons with gait speed less than 0.8 m/s are considered slow, which correlates with increased risk of falls.

Chapter 15

45. https://psnet.ahrq.gov/primer/falls/

46. E. Ekstrom, et. al. *Coordinated Care Plan to Prevent Older Adult Falls.* Edition 1.1. Atlanta, GA: National Center for Injury Prevention and Control, Centers for Disease Control and Prevention, 2021. https://www.cdc.gov/steadi/pdf/Steadi-Coordinated-Care-Plan.pdf

47. https://www.rehabmart.com/caregiver-university/.

48. https://www.skechers.com/

Chapter 16

49. https://www.gutenberg.org/ebooks/12

50. Matthew Lieberman. "Joe Lieberman Lived Life 110% to the End:, *Wall Street Journal,* April 11, 2024.

51. Roberts, A. (2018). Churchill: walking with destiny, Viking, Chicago.

ABOUT THE AUTHOR

Dr. Gradman received his MD degree from Harvard Medical School. He did his post-graduate training in general and vascular surgery at Cedars-Sinai Medical Center in Los Angeles where he practiced vascular surgery for over forty years before retiring in 2018. He received the Teacher of the Year Award in 1998. Currently, he lives in Beverly Hills with Susan, his wife for over fifty years, and he loves to play classical piano, travel, and dote on his three grandchildren.

Printed in Dunstable, United Kingdom